Academic Medicine - New Trends and Developments for the 2030s

Edited by Stanislaw P. Stawicki

Published in London, United Kingdom

Academic Medicine - New Trends and Developments for the 2030s
http://dx.doi.org/10.5772/intechopen.1005929
Edited by Stanislaw P. Stawicki

Contributors
Abirlal Sen, Antoinette Leonard-Jean Charles, Daryl O. Traylor, Davis Mendel, Eboni E. Anderson, Edie L. Sperling, Jennifer M. Hulett, Kevlian Andrew, Manidipa Barman, Mary C. Maj, Nikos Christo Secchi Nicolás, Sarjubala Thingujam, Sharmila Upadhya, Stanislaw P. Stawicki, Valerie A. Ubbes, Ángel de Jesús Gómez Alarcón

First published in London, United Kingdom, 2025 by IntechOpen
IntechOpen is the global imprint of INTECHOPEN LIMITED, registered in England and Wales, registration number: 11086078, 167-169 Great Portland Street, London, W1W 5PF, United Kingdom

For EU product safety concerns: IN TECH d.o.o., Prolaz Marije Krucifikse Kozulić 3, 51000 Rijeka, Croatia, info@intechopen.com or visit our website at intechopen.com.

British Library Cataloguing-in-Publication Data
A catalogue record for this book is available from the British Library

Academic Medicine - New Trends and Developments for the 2030s
Edited by Stanislaw P. Stawicki
p. cm.
Print ISBN 978-0-85466-017-9
Online ISBN 978-0-85466-016-2
eBook (PDF) ISBN 978-0-85466-018-6

Meet the editor

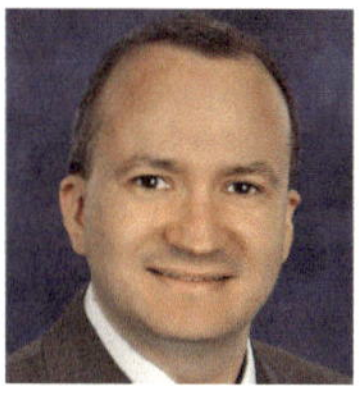

Dr. Stawicki is a Professor of Surgery and Chair in the Department of Research and Innovation at St. Luke's University Health Network in Bethlehem, Pennsylvania, USA. A specialist in General Surgery and Surgical Critical Care, he has co-authored more than 700 scholarly works, including over 30 books. Dr. Stawicki is recognized for his multiple national and international leadership roles in medicine. He is a member of numerous editorial boards and has been ranked among Stanford's Top 2% Scientists globally. His areas of expertise include artificial intelligence and machine learning in medicine, blockchain technology, patient safety, academic leadership, medical education, mentorship and coaching, traumatology and surgical critical care, and point-of-care sonography.

Contents

Preface

Dating back to ancient civilizations around the world, medical education has become the foundation for the sustainable transmission of knowledge and skills required to heal the sick, treat the injured, and promote overall well-being. Over the past two centuries, medical education has undergone significant expansion, accompanied by a growing understanding and the ability to treat a wide range of acute and chronic medical and surgical conditions. Beginning in the second half of the 20th century, the pace of medical progress and unprecedented aggregation of new knowledge resulted in the amalgamation of various academic medical pursuits into what we know today as "academic medicine", a unique blend of education, leadership, research, and clinical excellence.

Modern academic medicine continues to rapidly evolve as technological advancements and an expanding knowledge base combine to create new and unique opportunities and synergies. The pace and the highly dynamic nature of growth across all disciplines of medicine mandate that institutionalization of change becomes the new norm. The traditional "static ways" are no longer able to keep up with the real-time developments taking place.

Academic medicine cannot exist without a dedicated group of champions, or academic faculty. Traditionally, the idealized academic faculty member is considered to be a "triple threat", a term that refers to mastery of the primary areas of clinical care, teaching, and research. This concept has been evolving more recently, with some controversy surrounding the overly broad scope of the three core areas, resulting in the formation of "faculty tracks" (e.g., educator track, research track, clinical track, and, more recently, a leadership track).

It is anticipated that over the next 5-10 years, a truly impressive transformation will occur in the field of evidence-based medicine. Synergies resulting from the combination of accelerated creation of new medical knowledge and rapid technological advancements will enable faster and more effective ways of reviewing, verifying, and implementing clinical data. Natural evolution of this progress may help facilitate the emergence of evidence-based "smart curricula" and bias-resistant standardized assessments, as well as the implementation of "dynamic" evidence-based clinical practice guidelines, featuring near-real-time updates, clinical validation, and continuous improvement. As a result, diagnostic and therapeutic recommendations can be updated in real-time, with an emphasis on maximizing patient outcomes while optimizing resource utilization.

Equitable access to medical education remains a challenge worldwide, with various socio-economic factors, infrastructural considerations, and institutional credentialing barriers (e.g., entry requirements) hindering progress. This, in turn, represents a significant barrier to universal access to care, public health and well-being, especially in low-resource and rural environments. Modern technological developments, such as remote presence and AI-based educational platforms, may facilitate the gradual transition from classroom-centric to learner-centric approaches, overcoming the impediments of the traditional academic medical system, while maintaining the highest educational and accreditation standards.

Academic medicine's primary mission is to provide the backbone for the growth and development of the future generations of physicians. In addition to the key aspects already discussed above, the ability to provide a realistic simulation environment is another important tool that has been associated with improved real-life scenario performance and enhanced situational awareness across various clinical settings. Additionally, augmented reality holds promise to enhance everyday clinical experiences and workflows, particularly in the procedural realm. Other advantages of augmented reality may include better patient engagement and more effective remote consultations. Associated domains of research and development, especially in the area of patient engagement, include gamification and telerehabilitation.

Academic medicine should cultivate its focus on developing medical leaders with skill sets applicable to both academic and non-academic settings. Regardless of the composition of governing structures across different healthcare institutions, physicians who possess the required qualifications and administrative skills must provide key input into institutional decision-making processes. Consequently, leadership development and organizational engagement at various organizational levels and functional units, including medical education leadership, should be a key outcome measure of any successful academic medical program.

It is a sign of complacency to consider that the current academic medical system is somehow immutable. Across the globe, but especially in high-income countries, modern academic medicine represents a manifestation of the resources that enable or facilitate the evolution of fundamental clinical functions beyond the patient's bedside. Thus, significant reductions in financial support for the healthcare system will inherently translate into threats to various aspects of medical academics. In addition to navigating the rapidly changing landscape of artificial intelligence adoption and implementation, modern academic medicine also needs to address other pressing issues, such as scientific integrity, plagiarism, conflict of interest, and other types of misconduct, all of which potentially undermine the public's trust. This also extends into the realm of social media, with a significant risk of medical misinformation dissemination and potential downstream consequences.

In summary, academic medicine is a noble discipline within the modern healthcare paradigm. It is essential to the innovation and generation of new knowledge, the sustainment of our civilizational progress, and the preservation of knowledge, skills, and traditions accumulated over the millennia of the collective global "history of medicine" as it grew and evolved into its modern form. The next decade promises to be a time of great transition and opportunity for academic medicine. There are many areas of positive and exciting development, but there are also areas of concern and potential threats. It is the responsibility of medical academicians across all medical and surgical specialties, to ensure that the next generations of physicians are provided with a solid foundation for professional growth and development, from state-of-the-art medical education to cutting-edge leadership development opportunities. No matter the challenge, an unwavering commitment to the principles of ethical and human-centric frameworks must be maintained, regardless of any other factors and considerations.

Stanislaw P. Stawicki, MD, MBA, FACS, FAIM
Department of Research and Innovation,
St. Luke's University Health Network,
Bethlehem, Pennsylvania, USA

Section 1

Introduction

Chapter 1

Introductory Chapter: Transforming Academic Medicine of the Next Decade and Beyond

Stanislaw P. Stawicki

1. Introduction

Dating back to the ancient China, Egypt, Greece, India, and other early civilizations, medical education became the foundation of sustainable transmission of knowledge and skills required to heal the sick, treat the injured, and promote well-being [1–8]. During the late nineteenth century and throughout the twentieth century, medical education saw significant expansion, corresponding to the growing awareness of the importance of health and our growing ability to modulate various acute and chronic medical and surgical conditions [9–11]. Following World War II, the medical community around the globe saw a true renaissance within medical sciences, including the growth of organized, systematic approaches toward drug discovery, innovation, and evidence-based paradigms in general [11–14]. These new capabilities and perspectives gradually amalgamated into what became known as "academic medicine"—a unique blend of education, leadership, research, and clinical excellence [15–18].

Today, academic medicine continues to rapidly evolve as technological improvements and knowledge base growth combine to create and drive never-before-seen opportunities and synergies [19, 20]. In fact, the pace and the truly dynamic nature of growth within academic medicine mandates that "dynamic adoption," "empathetic change," and "adaptive assessment" become the new way, as opposed to the current, more static "periodic re-assessment and update" model [21–24]. Part of this transformation is the potential for technology-enabled decentralization of academic medicine and education in general [25]. Key concepts discussed in this chapter include the evolution of our current understanding of "academic medicine" as a distinct and unique entity, future opportunities for growth within academic medicine, as well as various controversies and potential threats pertaining to this broad topic area.

2. The "triple threat" is evolving

Traditionally defined and understood, the term "triple threat" refers to an academic faculty member who excels in three primary areas: clinical care, teaching, and research [26, 27]. This idealized paradigm envisions physicians who are not only skilled clinicians but also active researchers, effective educators, and often institutional leaders [26]. The concept has been evolving more recently, with some degree of controversy associated with the overly diluted focus areas, resulting in a tendency to form faculty tracks (e.g., educator track, research track, clinical track). This latter trend toward specialization is likely a reflection of the challenges associated with a single individual being the proverbial "Jack or Jill of all trades, master of none"—something that has become evident as the complexity of modern subdomains within the traditional "triple threat" definition became prohibitively high for a single individual to truly master [28, 29]. Additional focus areas have been introduced into the mix over the past few decades, including specialized tracks in medical leadership and academic international medicine/global health [30–34]. Dedicated advanced educational degrees have become more common among faculty members pursuing specific specialty areas / tracks [35–38].

3. Enhanced evidence-based approaches

Over the next 5–10 years, an impressive transformation will be taking place in the area of evidence-based medicine, across the entire spectrum of constituent factors—from clinical and scientific evidence generation to evidence-based medicine implementations [39, 40]. Highly effective synergies of multiple factors working together to produce amplification of benefits appear to be more of a question of "when" and not "if"—especially when it comes to timeliness of clinical data review, verification, and corresponding actionable implementations [41, 42]. Reinforcing the theme of "work smart, not hard" [43, 44], the introduction of machine learning (ML) and artificial intelligence (AI) technologies creates a unique opportunity to build significantly more efficient evidence-based "smart curricula" and bias-resistant standardized assessments [25, 45]. In addition, it will be possible to update and implement "dynamic" evidence-based clinical practice guidelines—a cornerstone of modern evidence-based practice—in a way that always includes the most recent scientifically and clinically validated data [41, 42]. Under such paradigm, diagnostic and therapeutic recommendations could be updated in near-real-time, with emphasis on maximizing patient outcomes while optimizing resource use. Similarly, validation and quality improvement processes within healthcare will also be amenable to analogous approaches.

4. Bringing school (and medical education in general) to the students

Access to medical education continues to be relatively restricted across the world—a combination of stringent prerequisites needed for qualified applicants and various resource-related factors (e.g., high cost of medical education, limited number of accredited educational institutions, and the requirement for ample technological and economic resources) [46–48]. This, in turn, represents a significant barrier to patient access to care and the ability to maintain public health and well-being at resource levels expected by the society, especially across low-resource and rural environments [49–52]. In this context, modern technological developments, including remote presence equivalent to in-person presence and AI-based educational platforms, enable the gradual transition from classroom-centric approach(es) to learner-centric approach(es) [25]. Within this new paradigm, traditionally understood "medical school" becomes a decentralized entity that is able to fulfill its stated mission while ensuring that highest educational and accreditation standards are maintained [25, 53, 54].

5. Immersive simulation and augmented reality

Academic medicine's primary mission is to provide the backbone for the growth and development of the future generations of physicians. The ability to provide realistic simulation environment has been associated with better real-time scenario performance across various clinical settings [55–58]. There is also evidence that "repetition is good" for both clinical pattern recognition and enhancing situational awareness [59–61]. Beyond educational settings, augmented reality promises to enhance everyday clinical experiences and workflows [62]. In the procedural realm, augmented reality promises to provide proceduralists with a more detailed and accurate intraoperative view of a patient's anatomy, contributing to less invasive surgeries and downstream benefits such as faster recovery times [63, 64]. Other advantages of augmented reality may include better patient engagement and more effective remote consultations [65–68]. Closely associated areas of research and development, especially in the area of patient engagement, include gamification and telerehabilitation [68].

6. Focus on leadership pipeline development

It is imperative that academic medicine maintains its focus on fostering the development of medical leaders, with skill sets applicable both in academic and in non-academic settings [69–71]. Associated skill sets include a variety of specific knowledge-based items (e.g., financial management, human resources management, regulatory frameworks) [17, 72, 73] and different so-called "soft skills" (e.g., emotional intelligence, coping intelligence, conflict resolution) [72, 74, 75]. It is generally accepted that the top-performing, top-ranked medical institutions are physician-led and rely heavily on physicians for leadership talent pipeline development [76–78]. That said, no statement is "absolute," and there are multiple excellent and successful non-physician-led healthcare organizations [79, 80]. Regardless of the constitution of the governing structures across different healthcare institutions, it is imperative that physicians who possess required qualifications and administrative skills provide key input into operational decision-making. It has been acknowledged by some in the relatively recent past that physicians and/or their time have been viewed increasingly as medical "content experts," and in some more recent publications, as "very expensive commodities" akin to professional athletes [81–83]. It is arguably a failure of the global medical education system, especially in high-income countries, to permit such a *status quo*. Consequently, leadership development and organizational engagement at various organizational levels and functional units, including medical educational leadership, should be a stated outcome measure of any successful academic medical program [84, 85].

7. Ensuring trainee, faculty, and staff well-being

The terms burnout, emotional exhaustion, and moral injury have become all-too-prevalent in the past decade, especially following the once-in-a-century event of Coronavirus Disease 2019 (COVID-19) pandemic [59, 86, 87]. It is now well-established that stakeholder participation in medicine in general, and academic medicine in particular, can be both physically and emotionally taxing [88–90]. Consequently, modern academic medicine must set among its many goals the emphasis on stakeholder mental and physical well-being. Lack of such emphasis will continue to contribute to the ongoing attrition and lack of sustainability, thus leading to suboptimal health outcomes for patient populations across the globe. By extension, the focus on personal well-being, again both physical and emotional, should be incorporated into medical school curricula during the earliest possible phases and subsequently reinforced throughout medical education, residency, and fellowship training and finally throughout one's professional career [91–93]. Benefits of such comprehensive approach are not only confined to the providers' well-being but also evident in better, more compassionate patient care and improved clinical outcomes [86, 90, 94–96].

8. Important pitfalls and threats

Although it is difficult to imagine the healthcare world without academic medicine and the many benefits it "brings to the table," one must not assume that the current place and function of medical academics as we know it can be taken for granted [97–99]. Across the globe, but especially in high-income countries, modern academic medicine represents a manifestation of resource levels that allow or facilitate the evolution of fundamental clinical functions (e.g., patient-centric clinical care delivery) beyond the patient bedside [16, 100–102]. Consequently, drastic reductions in financial support for the healthcare system will inherently translate into threats to various aspects of medical academics. Another potential longer-range threat to academic medicine is the risk of mismanaged introduction of artificial intelligence into our healthcare systems. More specifically, permitting artificial intelligence-based systems to assume various duties and responsibilities that currently are within the scope of academic faculty could potentially result in gradual erosion of knowledge and skills to sustain and maintain academic medicine as a unique area of expertise [103, 104]. Same can be said about complacent approaches toward developing knowledge, roles, and skills required to master artificial intelligence applications among academic faculty [105, 106]. Increasingly, medical academicians are also forced to navigate the highly complex ethical landscape of our modern academic healthcare [107]. Issues of scientific integrity, plagiarism, conflict-of-interest, and other types of misconduct threaten to undermine the public's trust in academic healthcare institutions [107–109]. Social media and the associated lack of content verification can lead to significant medical misinformation, potentially seeding further public distrust toward academic medicine [110–114]. Of course, there are many other potential modern threats to academic medicine—a topic that is out of scope for this introductory chapter—and the reader is referred elsewhere for further information [97, 98, 115, 116].

9. Synthesis and conclusions

Academic medicine is a noble undertaking within our overall modern healthcare construct. It is essential to the innovation and generation of new knowledge, the sustainment of our civilizational progress, and the preservation of knowledge, skills, and traditions accumulated over the millennia of the collective global "history of medicine" as it grew and evolved into its modern form. The next decade promises to be a time of great transition and opportunity for academic medicine. There are many areas of positive and exciting development, but there are also areas of concern and potentially even some threats. It is the responsibility of medical academicians, across all medical and surgical specialties, to ensure that the next generations of physicians are provided with a solid foundation for professional growth and development, from state-of-the-art medical education to cutting-edge leadership development opportunities. As always, an unwavering commitment to the principles of ethical and human-centric frameworks must be maintained, regardless of any intrusions of modern technological advances into medicine, inclusive of artificial intelligence.

Author details

Stanislaw P. Stawicki
Department of Research and Innovation, St. Luke's University Health Network, Bethlehem, PA, USA

*Address all correspondence to: stawicki.ace@gmail.com

References

[1] Elendu C. The evolution of ancient healing practices: From shamanism to Hippocratic medicine: A review. Medicine. 2024;**103**(28):e39005

[2] Tountas Y. The historical origins of the basic concepts of health promotion and education: The role of ancient Greek philosophy and medicine. Health Promotion International. 2009;**24**(2):185-192

[3] Engs RC. Health and Medicine through History: From Ancient Practices to 21st-Century Innovations [3 Volumes]. USA: Bloomsbury Publishing; 2019

[4] Harust YV, et al. Medicine and Humankind since Ancient Times: Historical and Legal Aspects of Joint Development. Ukraine: Sumy University; 2020. Available from: https://essuir.sumdu.edu.ua/bitstream/123456789/82626/1/Harust_%20Medicine_and_Humankind_%20since_2020.pdf

[5] Efthymiou-Egleton I. Wellness: A New Word for Ancient Ideas. Bloomington, Indiana, USA: Xlibris Corporation; 2017

[6] Ackerknecht EH. A Short History of Medicine. Baltimore, Maryland, USA: Johns Hopkins University Press; 2016

[7] Drabkin I. Medical education in ancient Greece and Rome. Academic Medicine. 1957;**32**(4):286-296

[8] Keswani NH. Medical education in India since ancient times. In: The History of Medical Education: An International Symposium Held February 5-9 1968. Oakland, California, USA: University of California Press; 2021

[9] Ludmerer KM. Time to Heal: American Medical Education from the Turn of the Century to the Era of Managed Care. Oxford, United Kingdom: Oxford University Press; 1999

[10] Fulton JF. History of medical education. British Medical Journal. 1953;**2**(4834):457

[11] Institute of Medicine, Board on Health Sciences Policy, Committee on Advancing Pain Research, Care, and Education. Relieving Pain in America: A Blueprint for Transforming Prevention, Care, Education, and Research. Washington, DC, USA: National Academies Press; 2011

[12] Claridge JA, Fabian TC. History and development of evidence-based medicine. World Journal of Surgery. 2005;**29**(5):547-553

[13] Roos R. Healing Milestones: Charting Medicine's Remarkable Voyage Through Time. Berlin, Germany: epubli; 2023

[14] Drisko JA. The history and evolution of medicine. In: Integrative and Functional Medical Nutrition Therapy: Principles and Practices. Cham, Switzerland: Springer; 2020. pp. 3-16

[15] Behrns KE. Transforming excellence in academic medicine. Missouri Medicine. 2018;**115**(3):203

[16] Konstam MA et al. The academic medical system: Reinvention to survive the revolution in health care. Journal of the American College of Cardiology. 2017;**69**(10):1305-1312

[17] de Guzman Strong C, Cornelius LA. Preparing the next generation in academic medicine: Recruiting and retaining the best. Journal of Investigative Dermatology. 2012;**132**(3):1018-1025

[18] Christmas C et al. Clinical excellence in academia: Perspectives from masterful academic clinicians. In: Mayo Clinic Proceedings. Philadelphia, Pennsylvania: Elsevier; 2008

[19] Reilly JB et al. Breaking down silos between medical education and health systems: Creating an integrated multilevel data model to advance the systems-based practice competency. Academic Medicine. 2024;**99**(2):146-152

[20] Khafizova AA et al. The impact of healthcare digitalization on the medical education curricula and programs: Points of convergence and divergence. Contemporary Educational Technology. 2023;**15**(4):ep479

[21] Haynes DM, Bonous-Hammarth M. Building a learning community for organizational change. In: Cultivating Equitable and Inclusive Conversations in Higher Education. Routledge; 2025. pp. 13-29

[22] Jia K et al. Constructing an empathy education system: Values, principles, and approaches. Journal of Moral Education. 2024;**12**:1-29

[23] Zhao L et al. Trends in the dynamic evolution of corporate social responsibility and leadership: A literature review and bibliometric analysis. Journal of Business Ethics. 2023;**182**(1):135-157

[24] Saxena R et al. Precision, personalization, and progress: Traditional and adaptive assessment in undergraduate medical education. Innovative Research Thoughts. 2023;**9**(4):216-223

[25] Stawicki SP. What's New in Academic International Medicine: Artificial Intelligence in Medical Education—A Once-in-a-Century Opportunity to Achieve Rapid Global Parity. International Journal of Academic Medicine. 1 Apr 2024;**10**(2):43-46

[26] Carlson ER. The triple threat: The quintessential goal of faculty development. Journal of Oral and Maxillofacial Surgery. 2024;**82**(5):509-511

[27] Manabe YC et al. Resurrecting the triple threat: Academic social responsibility in the context of global health research. Clinical Infectious Diseases. 2009;**48**(10):1420-1422

[28] Merritt C. Jack of all trades, masters of one? The Western Journal of Emergency Medicine. 2017;**19**(1):7

[29] Wiegers SE. Jill (or Jack) of all trades, master of none? Journal of the American Society of Echocardiography. 2015;**28**(6):628-629

[30] Gorgas DL, Prats MI, Bahner DP. What's New in Academic Medicine? Can International Medicine be an Academic Track? International Journal of Academic Medicine. 1 Jul 2017;**3**(2):211-214

[31] Garg M et al. A comprehensive framework for international medical programs: A 2017 consensus statement from the American College of Academic International Medicine. International Journal of Critical Illness and Injury Science. 2017;**7**(4):188-200

[32] Peck GL et al. The American College of Academic International Medicine 2017 Consensus Statement on International Medical Programs: Establishing a system of objective valuation and quantitative metrics to facilitate the recognition and incorporation of academic international medical efforts into existing promotion and tenure paradigms. International Journal of Critical Illness and Injury Science. 2017;**7**(4):201-211

[33] Kelley WN, Stross JK. Faculty tracks and academic success. Annals of Internal Medicine. 1992;**116**(8):654-659

[34] Howell LP, Bertakis KD. Clinical faculty tracks and academic success at the University of California Medical Schools. Academic Medicine. 2004;**79**(3):250-257

[35] Cohen R et al. An update on master's degrees in medical education. Medical Teacher. 2005;**27**(8):686-692

[36] Sherman WF et al. The dual degree orthopedic surgeon: A survey of the trends, motivations, and perceived value of the master of business administration degree. Orthopedic Reviews. 2021;**13**(2):24384

[37] Stellman JM, Cohen S, Rosenfield A. Evaluation of a one-year Masters of Public Health program for medical students between their third and fourth years. Academic Medicine. 2008;**83**(4):365-370

[38] Turner AD, Stawicki SP, Guo WA. Competitive advantage of MBA for physician executives: A systematic literature review. World Journal of Surgery. 2018;**42**(6):1655-1665

[39] Grol R, Grimshaw J. Evidence-based implementation of evidence-based medicine. The Joint Commission Journal on Quality Improvement. 1999;**25**(10):503-513

[40] Subbiah V. The next generation of evidence-based medicine. Nature Medicine. 2023;**29**(1):49-58

[41] Gould JA et al. Artificial Intelligence in Healthcare: Considerations for Adoption and Adaptation in Academic Medical Settings. London, England: IntechOpen; 2024

[42] Stawicki SP et al. Introductory chapter: Artificial intelligence in healthcare—Where do we go from here? In: Artificial Intelligence in Medicine and Surgery—An Exploration of Current Trends, Potential Opportunities, and Evolving Threats. Vol. 1. London, UK: IntechOpen; 2023

[43] Manson SM. Personal journeys, professional paths: Persistence in navigating the crossroads of a research career. American Journal of Public Health. 2009;**99**(S1):S20-S25

[44] Mazzarello S et al. Publishing clinical research: Ten pearls for oncology trainees and junior oncologists. Current Oncology. 2015;**22**(1):e1

[45] Stawicki SP, Martinez-Baladejo MT, Ng-Pellegrino A. What's New in Academic International Medicine? Artificial Intelligence and Machine Learning is Here to Stay, Forcing Rapid Adoption and Adaptation. International Journal of Academic Medicine. 1 Jul 2023;**9**(3):117-120

[46] Erschens R et al. Association of professional pre-qualifications, study success in medical school and the eligibility for becoming a physician: A scoping review. PLoS ONE. 2021;**16**(11):e0258941

[47] Conway-Hicks S, de Groot JM. Living in two worlds: Becoming and being a doctor among those who identify with "not from an advantaged background". Current Problems in Pediatric and Adolescent Health Care. 2019;**49**(4):92-101

[48] Millan LR et al. What is behind a student's choice for becoming a doctor? Clinics. 2005;**60**:143-150

[49] Wang Q et al. What are the challenges faced by village doctors in provision of basic public health services

in Shandong, China? A qualitative study. International Journal of Environmental Research and Public Health. 2019;**16**(14):2519

[50] Volosovets O et al. Current challenges for the health care system due to the lack of medical staff and the continuous professional development of doctors. Wiad Lek. 2022;**75**(5 p1):1136-1139

[51] Schluger NW et al. Creating a specialist physician workforce in low-resource settings: Reflections and lessons learnt from the East African Training Initiative. BMJ Global Health. 2018;**3**(5):1-5

[52] Girma T et al. Establishing medical schools in limited resource settings. Ethiopian Journal of Health Sciences. 2016;**26**(3):277-284

[53] Mlambo M et al. Transformation of medical education through decentralised training platforms: A scoping review. Rural and Remote Health. 2018;**18**(1):1-16

[54] Talib Z et al. Medical education in decentralized settings: How medical students contribute to health care in 10 sub-Saharan African countries. Academic Medicine. 2017;**92**(12):1723-1732

[55] Harper A, Mustafee N, Pitt M. Increasing situation awareness in healthcare through real-time simulation. Journal of the Operational Research Society. 2023;**74**(11):2339-2349

[56] Elendu C et al. The impact of simulation-based training in medical education: A review. Medicine. 2024;**103**(27):e38813

[57] Liu JYW et al. The effects of immersive virtual reality applications on enhancing the learning outcomes of undergraduate health care students: Systematic review with meta-synthesis. Journal of Medical Internet Research. 2023;**25**:e39989

[58] Iqbal AI et al. Immersive technologies in healthcare: An in-depth exploration of virtual reality and augmented reality in enhancing patient care, medical education, and training paradigms. Journal of Primary Care & Community Health. 2024;**15**:21501319241293311

[59] Stawicki SP et al. Introductory chapter: A quest to transform graduate medical education into a seamless journey toward practice readiness. In: Contemporary Topics in Graduate Medical Education. London, UK: IntechOpen; 2019

[60] Stawicki SP et al. A seven-center examination of the relationship between monthly volume and mortality in trauma: A hypothesis-generating study. European Journal of Trauma and Emergency Surgery. 2019;**45**(2):281-288

[61] Wang AI, Hoang TT. Reaction vs. completeness in game-based learning: Comparing two game modes in a game-based student response system. In: Proceedings of the 11th European Conference on Games Based Learning. Reading, Oxfordshire, United Kingdom: Academic Conferences and Publishing International Limited; 2017

[62] Navab N et al. Action-and workflow-driven augmented reality for computer-aided medical procedures. IEEE Computer Graphics and Applications. 2007;**27**(5):10-14

[63] Charlet M. Surgery of the future: Harnessing the power of virtual reality and augmented reality. In: Leveraging Metaverse and Analytics of Things (AoT) in Medical Systems. New York, New York: Elsevier; 2025. pp. 125-145

[64] Elsakka A et al. Virtual and augmented reality in interventional radiology: Current applications, challenges, and future directions. Techniques in Vascular and Interventional Radiology. 2023;**26**(3):100919

[65] Dinh A et al. Augmented reality in real-time telemedicine and telementoring: Scoping review. JMIR mHealth and uHealth. 2023;**11**:e45464

[66] Hilty DM et al. A review of telepresence, virtual reality, and augmented reality applied to clinical care. Journal of Technology in Behavioral Science. 2020;**5**(2):178-205

[67] Velázquez JS et al. New augmented reality application for improving clinical education and patient-doctor interaction in remotely-assisted ophthalmology consultations. Virtual Reality. 2025;**29**(3):96

[68] Berton A et al. Virtual reality, augmented reality, gamification, and telerehabilitation: Psychological impact on orthopedic patients' rehabilitation. Journal of Clinical Medicine. 2020;**9**(8):2567

[69] Dash NR et al. Development of a framework of leadership in academic medicine (FLAM). Journal of Medical Education and Curricular Development. 2024;**11**:23821205241296976

[70] Servey JT, McFate T, Reamy BV. Academic medicine in the military health system: Problems and solutions for academic leadership development. Military Medicine. 2018;**183**(1-2):7-10

[71] Howard-Anderson JR et al. Strategies for developing a successful career in academic medicine. The American Journal of the Medical Sciences. 2024;**367**(4):215-227

[72] Lobas JG. Leadership in academic medicine: Capabilities and conditions for organizational success. The American Journal of Medicine. 2006;**119**(7):617-621

[73] Pronovost PJ et al. Perspective: Physician leadership in quality. Academic Medicine. 2009;**84**(12):1651-1656

[74] Taylor N et al. Facing adversity during graduate medical training: The concept of 'coping intelligence'. In: Contemporary Topics in Graduate Medical Education-Volume 2. London, UK: IntechOpen; 2021

[75] Stawicki SP. What's new in academic international medicine? focus on conflict resolution strategies as a critical skill for modern academic leaders. International Journal of Academic Medicine. 1 Oct 2023;**9**(4):177-179

[76] Angood PB, Falcone CM. Preparing physician leaders for the future. Physician Leadership Journal. 2023;**10**(4):1-9

[77] Stawicki SP, Firstenberg MS. Fundamentals of Leadership for Healthcare Professionals. Hauppauge, New York: Nova Science Publishers, Inc.; 2018

[78] Firstenberg MS, Stawicki SP. Teamwork in Healthcare. London, England: IntechOpen; 2021

[79] Gupta A. Physician versus non-physician CEOs: The effect of a leader's professional background on the quality of hospital management and health care. Journal of Hospital Administration. 2019;**8**(5):47

[80] Mkandawire CY. Hospital Outcomes Based on Physician Versus Non-physician Leadership. Minneapolis, Minnesota: Walden University; 2017

[81] Mirand AL et al. Explaining the de-prioritization of primary prevention: Physicians' perceptions of their role in the delivery of primary care. BMC Public Health. 2003;**3**:1-6

[82] Gunderman RB. Commodity or profession? Journal of the American College of Radiology. 2008;**5**(4):540-543

[83] Nading M. "Medicine is not business, health is not a commodity, physicians are not salesmen!" clinical labor and Ukraine's health reform. Anthropology of Work Review. 2021;**42**(2):93-107

[84] Servey JT, Hartzell JD, McFate T. A faculty development model for academic leadership education across a health care organization. Journal of Medical Education and Curricular Development. 2020;7:2382120520948878

[85] Steinert Y et al. A teaching scholars program to develop leaders in medical education. Academic Medicine. 2003;**78**(2):142-149

[86] Salen PN, Stawicki SP. Introductory chapter: Enhancing physician wellness to prevent burnout promotes clinician and patient safety. In: Contemporary Topics in Patient Safety-Volume 3. London, UK: IntechOpen; 2024

[87] DeCaporale-Ryan L et al. The undiagnosed pandemic: Burnout and depression within the surgical community. Current Problems in Surgery. 2017;**54**(9):453-502

[88] Prentice S et al. Burnout, wellbeing and how they relate: A qualitative study in general practice trainees. Medical Education. 2023;**57**(3):243-255

[89] Solms L et al. Keep the fire burning: A survey study on the role of personal resources for work engagement and burnout in medical residents and specialists in the Netherlands. BMJ Open. 2019;**9**(11):e031053

[90] Tolentino JC et al. What's new in academic medicine: can we effectively address the burnout epidemic in healthcare? International Journal of Academic Medicine. 1 May 2017;**3**(Suppl 1):S1-S2

[91] Ripp JA et al. Well-being in graduate medical education: A call for action. Academic Medicine. 2017;**92**(7):914-917

[92] Dunn LB, Iglewicz A, Moutier C. A conceptual model of medical student well-being: Promoting resilience and preventing burnout. Academic Psychiatry. 2008;**32**(1):44-53

[93] Khan A, Vinson AE. Physician well-being in practice. Anesthesia & Analgesia. 2020;**131**(5):1359-1369

[94] Wallace JE, Lemaire J. Physician well being and quality of patient care: An exploratory study of the missing link. Psychology, Health & Medicine. 2009;**14**(5):545-552

[95] Sapra R. Social and emotional skills for health professionals. Indian Journal of Health & Wellbeing. 2019;**10**:410-414

[96] Lindow R, Gisch M, Marchini L. The importance of compassionate care. Brazilian Dental Science. 2023;**26**(1):1-7

[97] Levine AS et al. Research in academic medical centers: Two threats to sustainable support. Science Translational Medicine. 2015;7(289):289fs22

[98] Shomaker TS. Commentary: Health care payment reform and academic

medicine: Threat or opportunity? Academic Medicine. 2010;**85**(5):756-758

[99] Steinmann AF. Threats to Graduate Medical Education Funding and the Need for a Rational Approach: A Statement from the Alliance for Academic Internal Medicine. Philadelphia, Pennsylvania, USA: American College of Physicians; 2011. pp. 461-464

[100] Wartman S. The Transformation of Academic Health Centers: Meeting the Challenges of Healthcare's Changing Landscape. Oxford, United Kingdom: Academic Press; 2015

[101] Fennerty MB. Academic medicine under managed care. Gastroenterology Clinics of North America. 1997;**26**(4):911-921

[102] Korn D. Reengineering academic medical centers: Reengineering academic values? Academic Medicine. 1996;**71**(10):1033-1043

[103] Scherer MU. Regulating artificial intelligence systems: Risks, challenges, competencies, and strategies. Harvard Journal of Law & Technology. 2015;**29**:353

[104] Aoun JE. Robot-Proof: Higher Education in the Age of Artificial Intelligence. Cambridge, Massachusetts: MIT Press; 2017

[105] Kuleto V et al. Exploring opportunities and challenges of artificial intelligence and machine learning in higher education institutions. Sustainability. 2021;**13**(18):10424

[106] Yu H. The application and challenges of ChatGPT in educational transformation: New demands for teachers' roles. Heliyon. 2024;**10**(2):e24289

[107] Huecker M, Shreffler J. Ethical Issues in Academic Medicine. Treasure Island, Florida, USA: StatPearls; 2025

[108] Snyder Sulmasy L et al. Ethics and academic discourse, scientific integrity, uncertainty, and disinformation in medicine: An American College of Physicians Position Paper. Annals of Internal Medicine. 2024;**177**(9):1244-1250

[109] Davey M, Kirchgaessner S. Surgisphere: Mass audit of papers linked to firm behind hydroxychloroquine Lancet study scandal. The Guardian. 2020;**10**:10

[110] Plaza M et al. The use of distributed consensus algorithms to curtail the spread of medical misinformation. International Journal of Academic Medicine. 2019;**5**(2):93-99

[111] Stawicki SP, Firstenberg MS, Papadimos TJ. The use of blockchain in fighting medical misinformation: A concept paper. In: Blockchain in Healthcare: From Disruption to Integration. Cham, Switzerland: Springer; 2023. pp. 225-239

[112] Papadimos TJ, Stawicki SP. Hannah Arendt's prognostication of political animus in America: Social platforms, asymmetric conflict, and an offset strategy. Open Journal of Philosophy. 2020;**11**(1):85-103

[113] Stawicki SP, Firstenberg MS, Papadimos TJ. The growing role of social media in international health security: The good, the bad, and the ugly. In: Global Health Security: Recognizing Vulnerabilities, Creating Opportunities. Cham, Switzerland: Springer; 2020. pp. 341-357

[114] Conti K et al. The evolving interplay between social media and

international health security: A point of view. In: Contemporary Developments and Perspectives in International Health Security. Vol. 1. London, UK: IntechOpen; 2020

[115] Deckers PJ. Academic medicine: As threatened as most would have us believe? Gynecologic Oncology. 1996;**62**(2):151-158

[116] Harvey HB, Weinstein DF. Predatory publishing: An emerging threat to the medical literature. Academic Medicine. 2017;**92**(2):150-151

Section 2

Fundamentals of Medical Education

Chapter 2

Collaboration in Health Professions Education and Practice

Nikos Christo Secchi Nicolás and Ángel de Jesús Gómez Alarcón

Abstract

Nowadays, health professionals are increasingly specialized in different areas of knowledge within the various professions, which is intended to care for a population that suffers from multiple diseases and that needs the care of several health experts. This situation is disadvantageous, since sub-specialization breaks down interventions and does not allow for comprehensive care that prevents adverse events due to lack of intervention; it is also economically unsustainable for the health system, which needs efficiency and sustainability of its resources. Collaboration between professionals is understood as the joint effort of different experts in health and social areas to provide quality care. However, at present, interprofessional education in the health sector has not advanced at the same pace as the needs of society, presenting disjointed, outdated, rigid study plans with a notable lack of coordination in competencies. To facilitate teamwork, it is essential to receive training in personal and communication skills, as well as to know the functions and competencies of each professional. The adoption of interprofessional collaborative practice is considered essential to improving the quality of care and patient safety in healthcare facilities. This requires that health professionals acquire these skills through a flexible process that avoids prejudices and conflicts, allowing them to make the best decisions in the cases presented, thus preserving their professional autonomy.

Keywords: interprofessional education, interprofessionalism, interprofessional collaboration, interprofessional practice, interprofessional clinical simulation, collaborative learning, interprofessional curriculum

1. Introduction

New approaches to the organization, production, and valorization of work in the health sector are demanding an increase in information, knowledge, and the development of innovations both in the management of educational strategies and in the execution of health services. The recognition of the importance of fostering more intense collaboration during the training of future professionals in the health field and its connection with work practices implies fundamental adjustments in the organization of work and in the perception of roles. This requires the implementation of mechanisms that strengthen interpersonal interactions and foster trust for technical cooperation that integrates institutions and services, all with the ultimate goal of improving the quality of care and attention received by patients and users.

Collaborative practice is defined as the interaction between health professionals, which allows knowledge and skills to work together, benefiting patient care. Collaboration between disciplines refers to the joint effort where different professionals in the health sector and the social field join together to address problems or provide services. Additionally, teamwork is considered as the participation of several professionals with a common objective, which in this context results in offering high-quality care that promotes a positive and adequate evolution of the patient.

Interprofessional education (IPE) is a pedagogical approach in which members or students of two or more disciplines related to health or social care interact in learning with each other. Currently, IPE in the health field has not advanced at the same pace as social demands, presenting fragmented, outdated, rigid curricula with a significant lack of coordination in competencies. This results in the training of graduates who do not know how to collaborate effectively in a team, lack recognition of the roles of other professionals, have weaknesses in interprofessional communication, and have limited technical approaches, a narrow perspective, poor leadership, and evident difficulties in offering continuous care to the person and their environment. It is therefore necessary and appropriate to rethink IPE in health, taking into account the opportunities for joint and mutual learning that interprofessional work provides.

Interprofessional training represents an essential challenge that must be addressed in health sciences programs, in order to restructure the knowledge and skills of future health professionals from various specialties. This will allow them to adapt to the new roles required of them in their daily practice. It is essential to establish interprofessional collaboration to alleviate the current crisis of health personnel and provide quality care that fits the contemporary health model. Interprofessional education is gaining increasing relevance as a strategy to enhance the competence of human resources in the field of health, improve the results obtained, and, ultimately, strengthen the health system. To do so, it is crucial to contribute to the core of knowledge in this area, facilitating the recognition and understanding of its conceptual and methodological foundations, with the aim of maximizing its impact.

2. Methodology

A documentary research based on electronic sources was carried out. To select the bibliographic documents, various databases, journals, and academic repositories were used, such as BVS, Cochrane, Elsevier, Journal of Interprofessional, Medisur, Observatoriorh, PAHO, ProQuest, Redalyc, Educateconciencia, SciELO, the digital academic repository of the University of Navarra, Journal of Multidisciplinary Healthcare, Journal of Interprofessional Care, International Journal of Integrated Care, and the Google Scholar search engine. A bibliographic study was carried out where the terms used were interprofessional education, interprofessionalism, interprofessional collaboration, interprofessional practice, collaborative practice, health team, primary care, hospital care, perception, barriers, benefits; all connected by the Boolean operator AND. The filters were defined for "articles," "systematic reviews," "medicine," and "health professionals;" and the period was established from the year 2000–2025.

3. Interprofessional health education

Interprofessionalism can be understood as the evolution of a practice involving diverse disciplines, characterized by a process in which professionals analyze and develop approaches in response to the needs of the patient, family, and the community in an integrated manner. Interprofessional education is defined as an essential aspect of health professionals being "prepared to work collaboratively," a fundamental dimension for establishing team cooperation to address local health needs [1]. It is described as a partnership between a group of health providers and a patient in a coordinated, participatory, and collaborative approach to shared decision-making regarding health and social issues. The World Health Organization defines interprofessional education as a teaching and learning method that brings together students from different professions to learn together, with the goal of improving collaboration and quality of care [1]. Interprofessional collaboration (IPC) is defined as the process by which diverse groups of professionals work together to impact healthcare, optimizing work interactions and procedures among healthcare professionals [2]. Evidence suggests that barriers to IPC can have negative repercussions on healthcare, patient care, and the services provided. In contrast, research on interdisciplinary outpatient sessions has found a favorable impact, resulting in reduced hospitalization time and overall costs. Another study revealed a decrease in the prescription of psychiatric medications during monthly multidisciplinary team meetings [2]. Based on these findings, the authors argue that practical interventions aimed at improving collaboration can improve the quality of care and patient health, although they suggest further research is needed.

IPE is defined as a training session where two or more healthcare and social welfare professionals learn interactively, with the aim of motivating different professionals to meet and exchange ideas to improve collaborative practice [3]. A study conducted in the emergency department showed that IPE contributed to improved workplace culture and patient satisfaction and reduced the number of errors [3]. However, studies have also been conducted where IPE did not influence healthcare processes. Therefore, they conclude that the effectiveness of IPE is uncertain and has limitations, recommending continued controlled studies with larger samples and more appropriate control groups. To address IPE, it is essential to begin by differentiating between the terms multidisciplinary, multi-professional, interdisciplinary, interprofessional, and collaboration: a discipline focuses its attention on the field of knowledge, while the term professional focuses on the individuals who carry out the care tasks, in this context related to health [4]. The prefix "multi" represents distinct areas of knowledge or professional practice that maintain independent relationships [5]. Although they may share common goals, they operate in parallel, with limited interaction, while the prefix "inter" symbolizes a relationship of interdependence, marked by collaboration between different fields, oriented toward a common objective. Regarding the concept of cooperation in the field of IPE, several authors suggest that collaboration requires at least two people from different specialties or professions who are willing to join forces to improve the care provided to patients, families, and the community [6]. This joint effort aims to reduce competition in power dynamics, as this can affect the quality of care. However, collaboration means that everyone maintains their professional independence and that the boundaries between different professions are recognized.

An analysis conducted in the United States at various primary care facilities indicates that teamwork is linked to better care for older adults, reflected in improved functional status and shorter hospital stays, which fosters a safe environment for maintaining good health in the community [7]. Additional benefits include reduced mortality rates, fewer medication prescriptions, and greater patient satisfaction. Furthermore, it is highlighted that collaborative work favors better treatment adherence, fewer appointment cancelations, and more efficient use of health services.

Regarding obstacles, the study mentions a lack of political and regulatory support, as these are sources of funding that significantly impact health care, limiting access and available resources [7]. The conclusion drawn from this study is that teamwork is an effective strategy for achieving favorable health outcomes, although certain aspects need to be optimized, and further research is needed. Another document addressing primary care teams, which include all healthcare professionals—physicians, nurses, and pharmacists—evidences that collaboration is essential for caring for patients with multiple pathologies [8]. Communication, respect, and understanding of each other's roles and responsibilities and a willingness to learn and train are the essential foundations that drive collaboration. Positive results were achieved in terms of patient satisfaction and job satisfaction among professionals.

The study, conducted with medical and nursing students, demonstrates that collaboration among diverse professionals contributes to superior patient care [9]. Research supports the benefits of cross-disciplinary collaboration, as it improves healthcare outcomes and allows for optimal use of available resources. Among the students' comments, one medical student stated: "It was an invaluable educational experience; working together allows you to appreciate what each person contributes." A nursing student commented: "I feel like I've gained so much more knowledge by collaborating as a team; it's fantastic to witness professionals united in patient care" [9]. The structure of this study fosters collaborative education, establishing roles and responsibilities that optimize communication among team members and collaborative decision-making. The publication, published in several intensive care units, describes teamwork as the formation of a unit that promotes effective communication, as well as optimal coordination and cooperation among its members [10]. Furthermore, a positive mindset, mutual trust and respect, and joint involvement in the decision-making process are vital. Among the difficulties encountered in implementing teamwork, the concept of "teamwork" is mentioned, as each professional has a different interpretation of it. Furthermore, the predominance of medical power complicates interaction within the team. The study participants emphasized that communication is a fundamental value based on dialog and active listening, which facilitates more effective and fluid communication [10]. They also emphasize the importance of collaboration and coordination for teamwork, proposing the establishment of common goals that increase the effectiveness of care. Among the benefits obtained by healthcare professionals are reduced stress, increased personal satisfaction, and enhanced professional development [10]. In summary, it can be stated that teamwork enhances the quality of care, providing effectiveness and comprehensiveness; it allows for a better understanding of each patient's needs, minimizing errors and promoting the best decision-making for their well-being. A decrease in the length of hospital stays and in the use of resources is also observed, which in turn reduces costs.

An analysis conducted in an internal medicine unit reveals that patients treated by teams with high levels of collaboration among their members report, through a survey, greater satisfaction, a sense of security, and better pain control compared to those treated by teams with minimal collaboration [11]. On the other hand, no clear relationship was found between collaboration and the length of hospital stay. Thus, we could conclude that teamwork increases patient safety, noting that many avoidable errors are due to a lack of communication and collaborative work among professionals [11]. Two studies comparing the attitudes of physicians and nurses in various hospital units show that collaboration between members produces more positive patient outcomes and demonstrates personal development among professionals [12]. A positive correlation is established between the quality of relationships between physicians and nurses. It is noted that nurses tend to be more willing to collaborate compared to physicians. Furthermore, the variation in collaboration levels in more specialized units, such as surgical wards or intensive care units, is highlighted.

The root cause of interprofessional collaboration problems is found in the culture and ideology of the professions, to which are added new generations who often socialize for the first time with the culture of their profession, finding obstacles between their own group and others and transmitting attitudes and behaviors through gestures, reactions, use of spaces, silences, forms of humor, decisions, and it is in this context where the first restrictions for future collaboration are established [13]. For this reason, it is recognized that, for an interprofessional collaboration model to be effective, it must influence at least two levels, as seen in **Figure 1**.

a. Socialization in educational institutions [14]: This occurs mainly within professional training schools, in the structure of the curricula, in the collaborative skills of the trainers, in the establishment of channels of collaboration and mutual identification with other institutions, and in the design of external training activities that involve interprofessional contact.

b. Evaluations in the work environment [14]: This is related to the ability to create evaluation instruments with a focus on interprofessional collaboration, where the evaluation does not only depend on individual actions but also include a multilevel analysis in which the work environment and the organization itself are also critically evaluated.

The most significant aspect of this approach to interprofessional socialization lies in its ability to cultivate an interprofessional identity, without abandoning monoprofessional identities, since socialization occurs at the same time with other groups, moving from a flexible individual identity in various directions, according to demands and situations [14]. Considering the expansion, evolution, and dissemination of information and communication technologies (ICTs) and the knowledge-based nature of the economy, the perspective of interprofessional education clearly goes beyond the conventional confines of training and practice in the health field [14]. This active

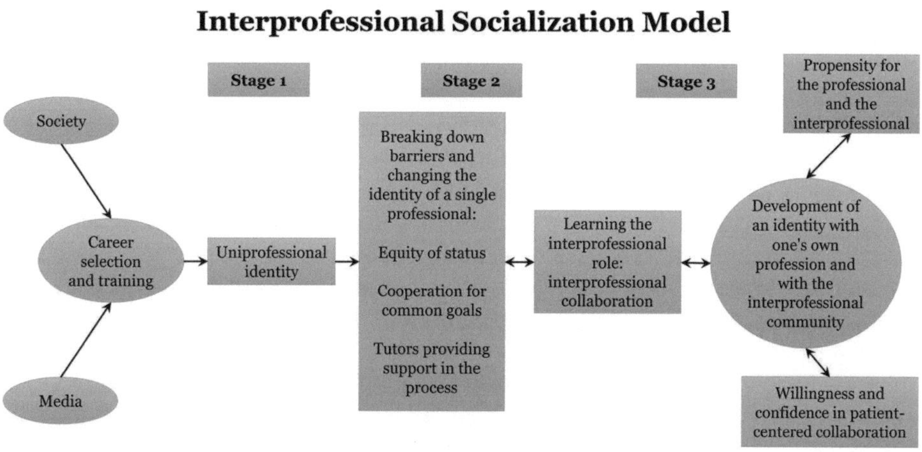

Figure 1.
Interprofessional socialization model. Source: Translated and adapted from Ref. [2].

perspective requires reevaluating and recovering previous training experiences, in addition to examining the interdisciplinary initiatives in the health sector that have driven organizational innovations, professional practice coordination processes, and social and community cooperation, all of which have been significant for its evolution and results. A historical connection can be found that merits analysis, since from this perspective, we can understand how the professional boundaries imposed by dominant knowledge have been crossed, enabling the current development of multiple shared and innovative actions in training and work among health professionals. Promoting a path toward interprofessionalism is an incremental process that encompasses various accumulation procedures, leadership development, and knowledge that support collective and institutional capital for the development of practices carried out by diverse professionals in the same or different health, social, and educational organizations [15]. This new knowledge is integrated and mobilized within daily work in different contexts. Interprofessionalism represents a multifaceted, dynamic, and sometimes contradictory opening when analyzing and reflecting on the impact of new health education strategies and their connection to social, economic, cultural, and epidemiological transformations within communities [15]. Achieving a comprehensive approach to collaboration among specialists is essential, as is establishing communication channels that materialize the application of interpersonal skills, fostering higher-quality care and attention.

In interprofessionalism, the professionals involved seek to agree on criteria through ongoing work, sharing information and knowledge, with the goal of analyzing and addressing a variety of educational and health problems with the participation of all stakeholders [15]. Thus, interprofessional education can be described as the process in which a group of students from diverse health-related professions, coming from different professional backgrounds, learn together by interacting over a specific period of their training, with the significant objective of collaborating in the promotion, prevention, treatment, rehabilitation, and other health-related services [15]. IPE aims to prepare students in health professions to provide high-quality care and attention through group strategies and practices developed in collaborative environments. Both interprofessional training and interprofessional practice are presented as processes that converge in the health field, as they foster joint learning between students and professionals in new practice environments. This process is understood as a field of articulation and exchange of knowledge and experiences that are planned, organized, and evaluated, with the aim of achieving a synergistic result for patient well-being and the resolution of health problems through collaborative dynamics [16]. The document entitled "Interprofessional Education in Health Care" by the Pan American Health Organization (PAHO) supports the need to adopt innovative approaches in the formulation of policies and programs that strengthen the health workforce globally, highlighting interprofessional collaboration as an innovative and promising strategy that contributes to addressing the global workforce crisis in this field [16]. In this context, collaborative practice in healthcare enables professionals from diverse backgrounds to provide comprehensive, high-quality services by interacting with patients, their families, and communities in all healthcare settings.

Interprofessional education and interprofessional practice do not contribute to improving health quality in isolation. Rather, their effectiveness grows within an institutional environment that fosters coherent and integrated care practices among professionals, thus facilitating effective communication to address health problems in response to people's needs, which contributes to a reduction in unnecessary interventions and overuse. Given the persistent lack of visibility of professional groups that have historically faced significant social inequities in health services, a secrecy that hinders true collaboration among professionals continues to persist [16]. This is because the knowledge and experience of one profession may not be valued by others, despite sharing similar scientific and clinical foundations and although skills and talents depend largely on individual backgrounds. Currently, there is an increase in the number of professions that have emerged following the scientific conceptualization of a body of knowledge. These professions, by specializing, fill gaps between existing professions, thus generating their own occupational space and demands [17]. Despite this, the secrecy and emotional and ideological loyalty toward the professional group to which one belongs remains palpable, such that closeness with members of other professions is discredited, considered a threat to the group culture that hinders authentic collaboration [17]. When the group implements collaborative practice, they show interest in each other's work, perspectives, and experiences; maintain communication with each other; assume interchangeable teaching and learning roles; and respond to each other until they form a professional identity in the exercise of their functions and healthcare [17]. It is crucial to transition from a professional identity (centered on oneself) to an interprofessional identity (centered on others) that focuses on the person receiving care. Interprofessional integration is shown below in **Figure 2**:

Therefore, the health system implements initiatives to enable health professionals to demonstrate their knowledge, skills, and attitudes in providing healthcare with a compassionate, ethical, safe, and people-centered approach. To this end, it focuses on the Global Competency and Outcomes Framework for Universal Health Coverage, issued by the World Health Organization in 2022 and encompassing the following competencies: (1) Person-Centeredness, (2) Leadership and Decision-Making, (3) Communication, (4) Interprofessional Collaboration, (5) Evidence-Informed Practice, and (6) Professional Conduct [17]. Interprofessional Collaboration impacts the following subdomains: (1) Collaborating with other healthcare professionals and patients; (2) Establishing and maintaining trusting relationships; (3) Learning from, with, and about other healthcare professionals and patients; (4) Constructively

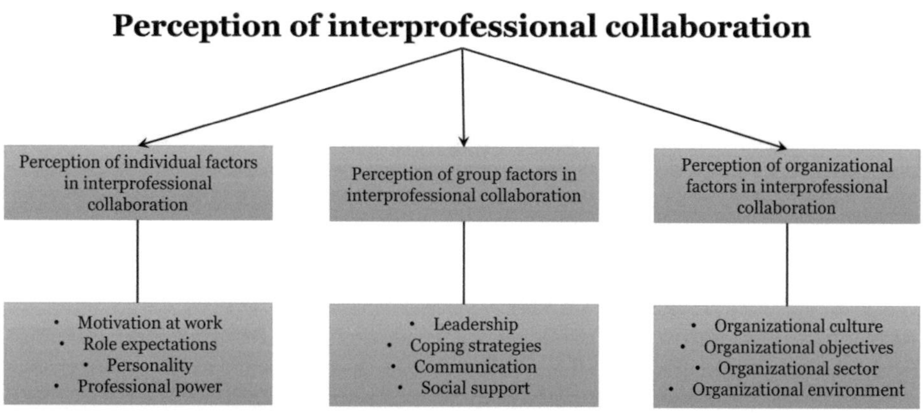

Figure 2.
Interprofessional integration. Source: Translated and adapted from Ref. [17]. Complete segregation = lack of contact between professionals. Interrelationships = exchange of information and referrals based solely on procedures and clinical guidelines. Network coordination = team without an individualized care plan. Cooperation = team based on an individualized care plan, which includes the role of a coordinator. Complete integration = collaboration that includes appropriate arrangements for the implementation of an individualized plan, co-financed by the authorities represented in the plan. For example, specific initiatives for individual care that include services such as accommodation provided by third parties.

addressing tensions and conflicts; (5) Evaluating individual and interprofessional team performance [17]. Considering that the healthcare team also includes professionals and trainees with diverse profiles from different educational institutions, it is suggested to implement a meaningful and cross-cutting Interprofessional Collaboration plan, tailored to the needs of the organization, through a concrete plan that can be gradually expanded according to circumstances and available resources. Currently, the transformation of health services is oriented toward actions such as the "managerialization" of the health sector, the "professionalization" of less-skilled occupational groups, the "specialization" of established professions, the "decentralization" of health entities in relation to the state structure, and the "participation" of users in the quality of services offered [17]. These five forces—managerialization, professionalization, specialization, decentralization, and participation—not only facilitate healthcare processes but also impact collaboration among health professionals, promoting a shift toward a teamwork model rather than a hierarchical organizational culture [17], as seen in **Figure 3**.

In 2010, the Interprofessional Education Office of the Faculty of Medicine and Health Sciences in Montreal, Canada, based its Interprofessional Education curriculum on the IPE competencies of the Canadian Interprofessional Health Collaboration Framework [18]. This framework encompasses a set of six competency areas that emphasize the growth of attitudes and behaviors, as well as values and judgments for collaborative practice. In 2011, the Interprofessional Education Collaboration (IPEC) of the United States presented the essential competencies, which were updated in 2016 [18], distributed among health professionals, and incorporated into the curriculum as well as accreditation standards, promoting the need to strengthen the Interprofessional Education and Collaborative Practice community, ensuring that this framework reflects the transformations in research, policy, and practice. The initial draft of the 2023 revisions of the IPEC core competencies for interprofessional collaborative practice is now available [18]. On April 3, 2022, the Global Competency Framework for Universal Health Coverage, a document developed by the World Health Organization that addresses the competencies required of health personnel to deliver healthcare was launched [18]. The competencies documented in 2010 (IHC), 2016 (IPEC), and 2022 (WHO) are shown in **Table 1** [18]:

The World Health Organization (WHO) maintains that Interprofessional Education and Practice is presented as an innovative approach that plays a crucial role in solving global health challenges [19]. However, it is also essential to carry out an examination and evaluation of the strategies that define both aspects, especially if it is considered as a mechanism capable of transforming the health system. From

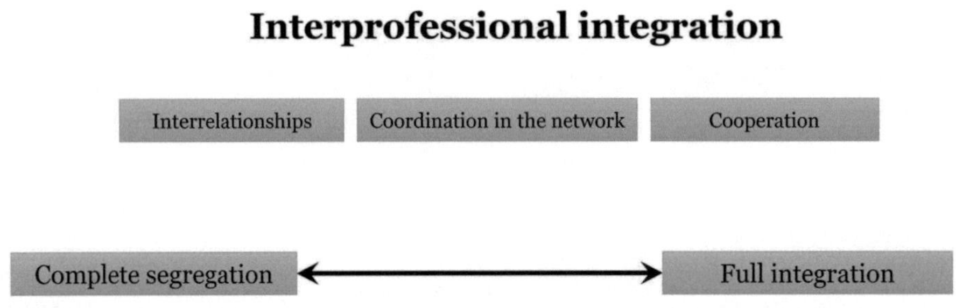

Figure 3.
Perception of interprofessional collaboration. Source: Translated and adapted from Ref. [2].

Canadian Interprofessional Health Collaborative Framework (CIHC), 2010	Interprofessional Educational Collaboration (IPEC), USA 2016	Competency Model for Health Personnel, WHO 2022
Patient-centered Care	Interprofessional Communication	People-centered
Collaborative Leadership	Teamwork	Decision-making
Interprofessional Communication	Ethical values for interprofessional practice	Communication
Team Functioning	Roles and responsibilities	Collaboration
Interprofessional Conflict Resolution		Evidence-based Practice
Role Clarity		Staff Conduct

Source: Own elaboration.

Table 1.
Documented interprofessional education competencies by CIHC, IPEC, and WHO.

this perspective, interprofessional education and practice should not be seen as independent activities that require additional learning. When a health team achieves a distinct configuration of professions and specialties, with clearly defined limits and a recognized and legitimized distribution of power, an interprofessional dimension is established at that moment [19]. Likewise, an improvement in quality is achieved by developing a varied and multiple set of sustained interventions over time. To do so, material resources, financing, continuing education activities, and adequate information through research are needed to draw conclusions and generalize results for decision-making. In higher education institutions, it is suggested to implement a clear IPE philosophy that influences the entire organization [20]. This philosophy must be known by the academic community and must be observable and measurable [20]. Faculty from various professions must collaborate in the creation of IPE learning experiences, integrating them into the curricula. In addition, it is essential to have an organizational structure that promotes IPE, which includes protected time for faculty to develop IPE strategies, incentive systems that motivate faculty participation, and joint activities between different health careers for students and faculty.

Interprofessional education acquires notable relevance as a strategy to strengthen the training of health personnel, in order to improve health outcomes, and, ultimately, strengthen the health system [21]. To do so, it is essential to advance in the understanding of this educational form that allows us to identify and understand its conceptual and methodological foundations. Health services are developed in response to this vision, as well as to the needs of communities and families, demographic and epidemiological changes, and social determinants, within a context of limited resources that force professionals to develop skills such as communication, conflict management, and innovation. Collaborative practice in the health field enables professionals from different specializations to come together to address problems and participate in decision-making, recognizing joint responsibility in achieving the expected results [21]. This allows for comprehensive care to be offered to patients, their families, and the community. In short, it is the joint effort of health professionals in the social field, aimed at solving problems or providing health services. For this reason, it is essential to promote the training of health professionals to collaborate in an interdisciplinary manner, ensuring effective interprofessional communication and coordination that involves key aspects such as trust, respect, and dialog among health workers [22]. Ethical values and principles that support authentic professional attitudes and appropriate interprofessional relationships must prevail. When experts collaborate in their work, the following elements occur simultaneously [22]:

1. Defined and common objectives in the care of patients and their families

2. Clarity in roles and responsibilities within the team: Each member performs his or her role with skill and innovation and also understands the obligations and tasks of other professionals.

3. Sense of group identity, empowerment, and mutual respect: Members feel part of the group and cohesive, trusting in the collective ability to face challenges and realize the shared vision.

4. Interdependence and integration in work practices between team members

5. Democratic approaches and collaborative leadership: Both the leader and the rest of the team recognize performance and success, both individual and group.

6. Initiatives to challenge stereotypes and obstacles

7. Time and opportunity to cultivate teamwork, separate from normal practice

8. Clear and unhindered communication: Differences of opinion and perspectives are valued.

The contemporary university has the task of promoting inclusive teaching among students from diverse professional profiles [23]. Therefore, modifications to the curriculum must focus on strengthening health systems and updating certain outdated pedagogical methods, in order to evolve toward systems that foster transformation [23]. This implies training leaders among students who become agents of change in their respective social-health environments. The advance in interprofessional education and practice invites us to rethink connections and to carry out research on the context in which it is developed, the sustainability of educational processes in the long term, and their impact on those involved [23]. It is necessary to examine experiences taking into account the processes of coordination, communication, interpersonal relationships, as well as both formal and informal power, in order to achieve interprofessional education and collaborative practice. The teaching foundations from which interprofessional education is proposed are [24]: The creation of knowledge is considered a collaborative and social task. Teaching is interpreted as an encounter that encourages the creation of connections and establishes an environment. Teaching is seen as a dialogic process, which entails reciprocity, participation, and interest. The teacher's position in teaching allows the student to occupy a central position. The teacher recognizes that in teaching not only content is transmitted, but it also communicates his personal experience with the content and his perspective on the students [24]. Considering that new learning is based on the student's prior knowledge, an essential task of the teacher is to help his group to review, question, and expand it. Teaching seeks the relevance of learning, so that students can connect what they acquire with what they already know. This is complemented by the social importance of the content [24]: what they learn can be applied to solve and analyze their professional life.

This is how teaching and learning are understood in a specific context. The beginning of teaching and learning is based on an aspect of life, not on a concept, nor on an abstract construction, nor on an explanation. It is taught from real situations of interprofessional work, which are significant in the real world [24]. Working with authentic situations facilitates the mobilization of knowledge and the commitment of students, giving space to the emergence of meanings related to its use in concrete practices. Teaching seeks to create challenges of interprofessionalism [24]. This involves posing situations that are challenging enough to force students to fully use their available knowledge, prompting them to question it again and develop novel ideas. This requires structuring activities that are slightly above the knowledge level of the students [24]. Teaching recognizes in the narrative approach the ability to promote processes of understanding and emotional connection with the content presented. Students are invited to reflect on their own thinking and that of others [24]. In this way, the class becomes an invaluable opportunity to reconsider one's own way of understanding. It can be said that teaching is intended to foster metacognitive processes that are crucial in interprofessional training. Education aims to promote deep understanding, since understanding, among other aspects, implies the ability to think and act flexibly based on acquired knowledge [24]. Therefore, knowledge is conceived not as something that is possessed but as an ability to apply it in different interprofessional contexts. Education values that the student plans and structures his or her own work. Education seeks to encourage the use of diverse sources of information. Education encourages the student to select modalities, methods, interlocutors, information sources, and so on. Education offers the possibility of enriching learning experiences by using a variety of resources.

It is essential to examine how a cooperation scheme fosters better integration in the health field [18]. Cooperation is not considered a temporary behavior; in recent decades of study, it has been shown that it reduces adverse events, improves safety, raises the level of satisfaction of health personnel, and optimizes the quality of the service provided. This clarifies that "the absence of collaborative practice between different professions can cause the patient to be exposed to the gaps that arise between areas of specialization [18]." **Table 2** below presents the terms that are most frequently related to IPE and **Table 3** with the advancement of interprofessional education in health.

The University of Toronto presents a model to foster core values and skills focused on Interprofessional Education in three stages [14]:

3.1 First level of development: Exposition

This level focuses on giving the student a first approach to reality and examining the interprofessional interactions that he or she will encounter in his or her future career [14]. Appropriate methodologies for this level could include:

3.1.1 Case analysis method

This technique is quite versatile; it can be an authentic case, an altered real case, or a fully devised one [25]. It is considered a fundamental activity in this phase of development, although it can also be applied in the immersion stage of the University of Toronto Model. Elements of a successful case are observed, where clear and direct situations are presented that provide practical and accessible solutions to promote the intuitive understanding of the participants, with a defined purpose to avoid deviations in the discussions and questions asked.

3.1.2 Analysis of film scenes

This resource is very valuable since film and television series clips during interprofessional sessions facilitate the creation of scenarios with non-verbal communication

Criteria	Multi-professional	Trans-professional	Interdisciplinary	Interprofessional
Staff	Two or more professions	Healthcare and non-healthcare professionals	Two or more health disciplines	Two or more professions
Interaction	No They learn or work together but do not interact with each other	Yes From your individuality	Yes From your individuality	Yes They learn, work, and interact
Role	Independent Parallel work, perhaps well-coordinated	Independent	Independent	They overlap (cover)
Scenery	Doctor preparing prescription Nursing preparing medicines Radiologist taking X-rays	COVID-19 vaccination campaign Firefighters Lawyers Engineers Managers Politicians Community leaders	COVID Hospitals Therapeutic plan for the Pulmonologist + Intensive Care Physician	Doctors and nurses coordinate to perform surgical procedures Communication between doctors, nurses, nutritionists, and psychologists in the treatment plan for a patient with DM

Source: Ref. [18].

Table 2.
Terms most related to IPE.

Undergraduate		Postgraduate			Teaching
Practical Activity		Competence			
Rookie	**Beginner**	**Competent**	**Professional**	**Expert**	**Teacher**
Didactic education, focused on the area of development, acquisition of knowledge and skills	Learning stage, supervised practice	Beginning of professional practice after obtaining and registering a professional title	Acquisition of operational skills through long-term practice. You may begin to gain specialist recognition	Maintains the highest level of knowledge, skills, and competencies, including leadership, vision, or recognition	Generates and maintains knowledge, skills, and recognition

Source: Ref. [18].

Table 3.
Progress of interprofessional health education.

and contextual analysis that are almost real and quickly assimilated. Another excellent alternative is the recording of videos for educational purposes [25].

3.2 Second level of development: Immersion

The objective of the immersion level is for the student not only to meditate on his or her relationships but also to begin to evaluate how to respond to these situations, experiencing and practicing [14]. Among the useful methodologies at this level, the following can be highlighted:

3.2.1 Simulation

Simulation is an extremely valuable tool that allows authentic situations to be recreated in the classroom, requiring adequate logistics. The repetition and practice of cases can be a little complicated, but it is a necessary addition to the development of the second stage of the University of Toronto model. It is an ideal and essential complement [25].

3.2.2 Role Playing

Role playing involves assuming a character, providing the opportunity to represent specific situations by acting out a previously determined role, where the participant makes decisions and shows his or her performance. Afterwards, a debriefing can be carried out with practical protocols that allow students to explore and experiment with structured ways of offering responses to various situations analyzed [25].

3.2.3 Virtual scenarios with avatars

Virtual environments are an exceptional tool for creating digital spaces simulating a kind of video game, where participants can react to different interprofessional situations in contexts as close to reality as possible, using their avatar, as could be the case in a hospital environment [25].

3.3 Third level of development: Competence

The level of competence seeks to have the student demonstrate the interprofessional skills acquired in practice situations that resemble real life [14]. Effective strategies at this level could include caring for real patients (whether in a hospital, community, or home environment) and remote care through telemedicine.

4. Teaching strategies

The most recognized educational methodologies for interprofessional education include case-based learning, problem-driven learning, clinical simulation, seminars, workshops, collaborative research, and online learning [18]. Online learning serves as either a primary or complementary strategy, being most effective when it supports face-to-face training. In any case, the tactics employed must be participatory and reflective, and their selection may change throughout the training process depending on several factors such as the topic, objectives, stage, professions, and context, among others [18]. It is essential to keep in mind that the strategies used are not limited solely to the presence of different professionals but must facilitate interprofessional interaction and cooperation [17]. A crucial point for the successful implementation of interprofessional education is that teachers need prior preparation to thoroughly understand the concept, objectives, methods, and strategies. This will facilitate effective interaction through workshops with teachers from other disciplines, also allowing them to learn about pedagogy and practice in other professions. It is vital to consider that they must receive ongoing support and advice. It is suggested that interprofessional education be delivered in small groups; however, large-group activities can be combined with smaller-group activities to maximize the use of resources. At the European University of Madrid, the classification of teaching strategies applied by level includes: at the exposition level [18], the most commonly used techniques have been case studies, problem-based learning (PBL), film sequence analysis, and reflective learning; for the immersion level, role-playing and simulation are used; and for the competence level, planning and healthcare delivery in real-life contexts by the interprofessional team are carried out.

Below are some educational strategies implemented in training programs that have incorporated interprofessional education:

4.1 Case-based learning

Learning based on integrative cases has become one of the most common methodologies within IPE [26]. This technique is carried out by presenting a case, either virtually or in person, allowing adequate time for students from various disciplines to discuss how to collaborate and find solutions based on the reflective questions posed. A study that reports the use of simulated patients and cases involving chronic diseases that require a multi-professional team was conducted by Orsini in 2019 [26]. In this study, students were required to assess patients, then discuss the information they had gathered as a group, and ultimately propose an appropriate treatment plan. Team collaboration and case resolution were assessed, with feedback received from both educators and patients involved.

4.2 Problem-based learning

Problem-based learning (PBL) has been used as an educational approach since the 1960s [25]. Its first implementations were at the Case Western Reserve University School of Medicine in the United States and at McMaster University in Canada [25]. PBL is a multi-methodological and multi-didactic educational model designed to motivate and facilitate the teaching-learning process and student development. This approach promotes self-learning, self-assessment, and self-regulation, processes that are enhanced by its dynamic approach and its constructivist vision. In PBL, students learn from problems that are relevant to them, using mistakes as another opportunity to learn. Working in small groups of no more than ten, this fosters the development of communication skills, interpersonal relationships, and collaborative teamwork. Several educational centers have implemented IPE based on problem-based learning. Two examples are presented below: At the University of Navarra in Spain, Interprofessional Education has been integrated into the curriculum through three elective courses delivered over three consecutive semesters, referred to as Interprofessional Education 1, 2, and 3 [27]. The first course identifies the competencies to be promoted and highlights the importance of interprofessional education through PBL. The second focuses on clinical simulation as a safe and controlled environment where students can learn from their own experiences. And the third focuses on real-life problem-solving in an interprofessional context, where students are grouped together to care for chronically hospitalized patients [27]. The competencies to be developed include interprofessional communication, team collaboration, respect for roles, and conflict resolution. All three courses reinforce the idea that success lies not in an individual but in the work of a group. On the other hand, at the Universidad de la Frontera in Chile, the Faculty of Health Sciences, aiming to respond to integrative and multidisciplinary approaches, carried out a project implementing a workshop called "Learning Skills Workshop" at the beginning of the educational process [28]. The purpose is to foster communication and collaboration skills and to understand perceptions regarding the advantages and disadvantages of PBL. This workshop lasts 12 hours and is structured into three units addressing communication, teamwork, small-group learning, and problem-based learning, each lasting 4 hours [28]. Students' perceptions of the benefits focus on contributing to the development of well-rounded professionals, with skills that enable them to meet current societal demands with a global perspective, such as teamwork, critical thinking, autonomous and continuous learning, integration of knowledge to solve health problems, a multi-professional approach, and self-assessment as a tool for personal development.

4.3 Reflective learning

There are various theories of reflective learning, among which those proposed by John Dewey, David Kolb, and Graham Gibbs stand out [29]. According to reflective learning theory, reflection is considered essential for people to evolve as human beings through their interaction with society. Without increasingly systematized reflection, there is no true learning, development, or education in human beings. Learning is not equivalent to simply knowing, repeating, or acquiring information in any way; it involves a reflective and abstract construction of experience, which gives this activity a very human uniqueness [29]. Kolb developed a complete learning cycle that highlights the importance of experience in the learning process, especially in situations considered critical incidents [30]. This cycle encompasses aspects of sensing, observing, thinking, and doing, beginning with a concrete experience that is subjected to reflection to generate abstract concepts, which are applied and verified in new situations. It is essential to incorporate emotions and their influence into actions and reflection [30]. The Gibbs Reflective Cycle provides a framework for analyzing experiences and, due to its cyclical nature, is particularly well-suited to repetitive experiences, allowing for learning and planning based on what went well or poorly; this methodology has been implemented in nursing program training [31].

4.4 Clinical simulation

Today, clinical simulation is used to develop the necessary skills and competencies in healthcare students. It promotes learning through concrete experiences, goal setting, practice, and reflection in comparison with previous theories, and, finally, conceptualizing what has been learned to solve problems and make decisions [32]. This fosters the desire to learn from new experiences and restart the cycle. Simulation has been shown to promote long-term learning, reducing the occurrence of adverse events in patients [32]. Combined with effective planning and analysis of results, it has facilitated the maintenance of good practices and the development of new solutions when faced with opportunities for improvement. Traditionally, simulation has been carried out with individuals from the same area, using role-playing in situations that warrant it; however, in the context of IPE, students can interact in the same situation with colleagues from different professions [32]. This will help them overcome their fears about interaction, gain confidence, clearly understand their role, and recognize the importance of working in an organized manner according to their professional scope without exceeding their responsibilities. Recently, several reports supported the effectiveness of training through high-fidelity simulations in healthcare and education institutions, integrating staff from multiple professions to develop teamwork skills, which are then transferred to real-life contexts and sustained in daily activities [32]. A reduction in the detection time of alarming signs and in the care provided has also been demonstrated.

4.5 Seminars

The seminars have fostered the establishment of educational spaces for the renewal and updating of important topics, approaches, and content for IPE [25]. They are considered one of the various institutional strategies for advancing the program, as indicated by the University of Arkansas in the United States and the University of Brasilia in Brazil [25]. At the Ceilandia campus of the University of Brasilia, the creation of an academic space dedicated to the renewal and updating of key topics, approaches, and content for training has been promoted. These seminars are organized regularly, typically per semester, and involve students from various professions, lasting approximately 30 hours [25]. The objective of the seminar is to systematize the content covered during the semester and enrich it through the contributions of the various participants, facilitated by challenging questions posed by a faculty committee. This committee, composed of professors from all professions, is responsible for defining the parameters for the seminar's implementation. Their role involves introducing complex topics that may generate concern or surprise, as well as encouraging in-depth analysis of issues of relevance to health education, which leads to the generation of diverse perspectives [25]. During the seminars, other academic activities are suspended to ensure sufficient time to focus on the presentation of results.

4.6 Collaborative research

Research groups are formed as spaces for the creation of knowledge, which supports the Interprofessional Education (IPE) approach [33]. Team activities are crucial and allow for an enriching exchange of experiences among participants. Since 2007, the Interprofessional Health Education Research Group at the Federal University of São Paulo, Brazil [33], has conducted studies and research in the field of interprofessional health education; promoted the production and dissemination of scientific knowledge; organized educational, pedagogical, cultural, technical, and scientific activities that interact with the academic community and society; and promoted and established reciprocal collaborations with both national and international centers, based on ethical and social principles [33]. In 2018, they published the findings of a qualitative research project that incorporated case study elements and was contextualized within a research narrative [33]. The analysis of the narratives concluded that the research group acts as an incubator, creating environments conducive to cultivating critical and reflective thinking and collaborative skills that engage its members in a constant cycle of action-reflection-action; it stands out as a privileged space for sharing, producing, and building knowledge grounded in interprofessionalism, maintaining horizontal relationships that also foster the establishment of networks around IPE, both within and outside the institution.

4.7 Online learning

The Universidad del Rosario, located in Colombia, launched an online course in 2019 for first- and second-semester students in speech therapy, medicine, occupational therapy, physical therapy, and psychology [34]. This interpretive qualitative analysis, which uses a deductive thematic analysis approach, examined the experience 6 weeks after its launch. Positive evaluative aspects included the relevance of the contributions to clinical case resolution, even when the students were in their initial stages, as well as commitment, respect, critical thinking, and the opportunity to learn about other disciplines [25]. Regarding areas for improvement, the need for faculty to dedicate more time, establish at least one in-person meeting, and provide greater clarity on the platform was identified. Online interdisciplinary education has been used primarily as a complement to other strategies, constituting an alternative to balance activities with the schedules established by the academic program. It can be effective in boosting student motivation [34]. Therefore, it should be developed by a multidisciplinary team with skills in multimedia design and development.

5. Advantages of interprofessional health education

By focusing interdisciplinary education on the patient, family, and the community from a comprehensive perspective, its main advantage is the efficiency and quality of care, which has been demonstrated by improved patient satisfaction with the care and information received [35]. Furthermore, time has been optimized because the work is carried out as an interdisciplinary team rather than each professional treating the patient in isolation. At the community level, the public perception of healthcare teams has improved [35]. The benefits for healthcare personnel include understanding of roles, changing attitudes, respecting and valuing everyone on the team, preparing for future interprofessional collaborations, increasing self-esteem and communication skills, facilitating information sharing, problem-solving, and applying knowledge from common and specific foundations [35].

The World Health Organization emphasizes its usefulness in reducing adverse events and published a multi-professional curriculum guide on patient safety in 2012 [25]. This guide consists of two sections: the first is intended for health science educators, and the second is intended for educators and students, covering in detail eleven topics related to policy and global challenges related to patient safety [25]. The guide was developed to facilitate its adaptation to different health training program curricula. Analyzing the impact of implementing the above guide in relation to its purpose of reducing adverse events, it can be deduced that this entails benefits both in patient recovery and in family satisfaction, in addition to reduced costs for institutions due to the mitigation of the consequences of such adverse events and the reduction of lawsuits and costly compensation claims [25]. In the health systems field, progress is being made toward an approach that prioritizes promotion and prevention rather than focusing solely on diagnosis and treatment. To achieve this, the importance of interprofessional teamwork and intersectoral efforts is recognized to reinforce the principle of comprehensiveness.

6. Difficulties and limitations in the implementation of interprofessional education in health

IPE presents difficult challenges to implement, as it entails complex processes such as: Systemic, which is related to factors external to the organization, including government policies and support from state institutions [36]; organizational, which refers to understanding the relevance of IPE from the perspective of the authorities of health training institutions and, consequently, how leadership is exercised and participation is achieved [36]; inclusion in the curricula or curriculum designs of the different programs, as it requires a thorough analysis to select topics, activities, methodologies, human and material resources, and training times, among others, that are consistent with the existing structure [36]; interaction, which involves leaving the comfort zone and seeking innovative strategies through the participatory approach of teaching teams from diverse professions, based on their motivation and willingness to collaborate, the way they communicate, and their ability to resolve internal conflicts [36]. Limitations have also been identified, such as the exercise of power, the hierarchization of professions, and the management of technologies in simulation or information and communication.

7. Conclusion

Interprofessional education is presented as a pedagogical methodology that ensures that students in the medical sciences are equipped to participate in collaborative practices that address patients' health problems. This form of education promotes an exchange of knowledge and roles among members of basic health teams, fostering effective communication between professions and respect for each other's roles in patient care. Currently, despite the multiple advantages that interprofessional education offers in undergraduate training in the fields of medical sciences, its implementation is not considered within the curricular design. Therefore, interprofessional education and practical collaboration should be fundamental when developing curricula in these disciplines. Such curricular designs must be relevant and establish the bases for a continuous increase in the quality and effectiveness of the comprehensive training of health professionals.

An organization seeking interprofessional training needs to integrate various institutional dimensions in macropolitical and micropolitical contexts, where interests, ambitions, and alliances with diverse orientations coexist. The need to address personal stereotypes leads to negotiations, renegotiations, and mediation processes to reach consensus in the face of conflicts that aim to place oneself in a favorable position in decision-making. In addition, the resources and willingness to collaborate in shared tasks cannot prosper without the creation of environments conducive to learning and teamwork. From this point of view, it is proposed to think and exchange ideas to build connections between different areas.

Today, it is essential in the health field to know and explore which situations promote and which limit interprofessional training in complex organizations, such as educational and health organizations. Providing answers to a variety of concerns and questions will allow the design of new educational strategies and the training of competent professionals through collaborative practices, recognizing that the main source of value in the current stage of health development is the knowledge acquired and mobilized by the active work of professional teams.

In recent years, strategies focused on joint learning, improved communication, and the development of skills in medical and nursing students have been implemented, which have shown positive results for both professionals and patients. Among the barriers that hinder collaborative practice, the most notable is the policy of each country, the system of organization in access to health, and current legislation.

Among the benefits that impact the patient, the increase in safety, the reduction in the length of hospitalization, patient satisfaction, and the optimization of costs and available resources stand out. It also favors the relationship between the different professionals, contributing to the development of their skills and to maintaining a good emotional state, which helps to effectively manage the stress caused by the work. It is essential to train health students at university and promote collaborative work. It is essential to invest time in prevention and health promotion, since preventing diseases before they arise can improve patient quality of life and allow savings in materials and resources. It is necessary to improve state policy to guarantee healthcare.

Author details

Nikos Christo Secchi Nicolás* and Ángel de Jesús Gómez Alarcón
Independent Researcher, Minatitlán, Veracruz, Mexico

*Address all correspondence to: drsecchi@hotmail.com

References

[1] Soto-Ruiz N, Escalada-Hernández P, Ortega-Moneo M, Viscarret-Garro JJ, Martín-Rodríguez LS. Educación interprofesional en ciencias de la salud con la colaboración de pacientes. Educación Médica. 2022;**23**(1):1-7

[2] Merrick Z, Joanne G, Scott R. Interprofessional collaboration: Effects of practice-based interventions on professional practice and healthcare outcomes. Cocharane Database of Systematic Reviews Cochrane Library. 2009;**3**(1):1-29

[3] Reeves S, Zwarenstein M, Goldman J, Barr H, Freeth D, Hammick M, et al. Educación interprofesional: Efectos sobre la práctica profesional y los resultados de la asistencia sanitaria. The Cochrane Library. 2008;**3**(1):1-41

[4] Amato D, Gómez-Clavel JF, Novales-Castro XJ. ¿Interdisciplinario o interprofesional? Investigación en Educación Médica. 2019;**8**(32):125-126

[5] Costa-Viana M, Filho-Rodrigues FJ, Silva-Brandão GC. Educación Interprofesional en Salud. Primera ed. Brasil: SEDISUFRN; 2018

[6] Peduzzi M, Agreli HF, da Silva JAM, de Souza S. Trabalho Em Equipe: Uma Revisitaao Conceito E A Seus Desdobramentos No Trabalho Interprofissional. Trabalho, Educacao e Saúde. 2020;**18**(1):1-20

[7] Solheim K, McElmurry BJ, Kim MJ. Multidisciplinary teamwork in US primary health care. Social Science and Medicine. 2007;**65**(3):622-634

[8] Dieleman SL, Farris KB, Feeny D, Johnson J, Tsuyuki RT, Brilliant S. Primary health care teams: Team members' perceptions of the collaborative process. Journal of Interprofessional Care. 2004;**18**(1):75-78

[9] Corbridge SJ, Tiffen J, Carlucci M, Zar FA. Implementation of an interprofessional educational model. Nurse Educator. 2013;**38**(6):261-264

[10] Del Barrio LM, Reverte SM. Evaluación del trabajo en equipo en seis unidades de cuidados intensivos de dos hospitales universitarios. Enfermería Intensiva. 2010;**21**(4):150-160

[11] Havyer RDA, Wingo MT, Comfere NI, Nelson DR, Halvorsen AJ, McDonald FS, et al. Teamwork assessment in internal medicine: A systematic review of validity evidence and outcomes. Journal of General Internal Medicine. 2014;**29**(6):894-910

[12] Thomson S. Nurse-physician collaboration: A comparison of the attitudes of nurses and physicians in the medical-surgical patient care setting. Medsurg Nursing: Official Journal of the Academy of Medical-Surgical Nurses. 2007;**16**(2):87-91

[13] Spaulding EM, Marvel FA, Jacob E, Rahman A, Hansen BR, Hanyok LA, et al. Interprofessional education and collaboration among healthcare students and professionals: A systematic review and call for action. Journal of Interprofessional Care. 2021;**35**(4):612-621

[14] Khalili H, Thistlethwaite J, El-Awaisi A, Pfeifl A, Gilbert J, Lising D, et al. Orientación para la investigación global sobre EIP.indd. Publicación conjunta de Interprofessional Research. Global e Interprofessional. Global; UW Center for Interprofessional Practice

and Education; University of Wisconsin-Madison; 2019. [Acceso 20 de Febrero de 2025]

[15] Frenck J, Chen L, Bhutta ZA, Cohen J, Crisp N, Evans T, et al. Health professionals for a new century: Transforming education to strengthen health systems in an interdependent world. Lancet. 2010;**376**(9756):1923-1958

[16] Organización Panamericana de la Salud. IRIS PAHO. 2017. Disponible en: http://iris.paho.org/xmlui/handle/123456789/34372 [Acceso 26 de Mar de 2025]

[17] Ayala R. Gestión del Cuidado Interprofesional. Santiago de Chile: Ril Editores; 2019

[18] Beunza Nuin JJ, Icarán FE. Manual de educación interprofesional sanitaria. Primera ed. Barcelona, España: Elsevier Health Sciences; 2018

[19] Dyess AL, Brown JS, Brown ND, Flautt KM, Barnes LJ. Impact of interprofessional education on students of the health professions: A systematic review. Journal of Educational Evaluation for Health Professions. 2019;**16**(33):1-6

[20] Zechariah S, Ansa BE, Johnson SW, Gates AM, Leo GD. Interprofessional education and collaboration in healthcare: An exploratory study of the perspectives of medical students in the United States. Healthcare (Basel, Switzerland). 2019;7(4):1-11

[21] Lajes Ugarte M, Aúcar López J, Martínez Morell A, Aguilar RY. El trabajo colaborativo interprofesional en el proceso de formación profesional en salud. Revista de Humanidades Médicas. 2021;**21**(3):951-966

[22] de Groot E, der Vossen M, Slootweg I, Çorum M, Kramer A, Muris J, et al. Advancing collaboration in health professions education in the general practice domain, developing a national research agenda. Advances in Health Sciences Education. 2024;**29**(1):1417-1434

[23] Díaz-Ortiz A, Durand-Rill R, Robinson-Jay F. La educación colaborativa interprofesional en los estudios de pre y posgrado en Ciencias de la Salud. Revista Información Científica. 2023;**102**:1-14

[24] Mohammed CA, Anand R, Ummer VS. Interprofessional education (IPE): A framework for introducing teamwork and collaboration in health professions curriculum. Medical Journal Armed Forces India. 2021;**77**(1):16-21

[25] Ferreira Parreira MS, Fernandes Agreli H, da Silva JAM, Rodrigues Freire Filho J, da Costa MV, Alves Batista N, et al. Educación Interprofesional en Brasil. In: Beunza Nuin JJ, Icarán Francisco E, editors. Manual de educación interprofesional sanitaria. Barcelona, España: Elsevier Health Sciences; 2018. pp. 115-135

[26] Bridges D, Davidson RA, Soule Odegard P, Maki IV, Tomkowiak J. Interprofessional collaboration: Three best practice models of interprofessional education. Medical Education Online. 2011;**16**(1):1-10

[27] La Rosa-Salas V. Educación interprofesional: una propuesta de la Universidad Navarra. Educación Médica. 2020;**21**(6):386-396

[28] Navarro N, Illesca Pretty M, Cabalín D. Experiencia multiprofesional de Aprendizaje Basado en Problemas. Facultad de Medicina. Universidad de la Frontera. Revista de Educación en Ciencias de la Salud. 2004;**1**(1):25-30

[29] González Calvo G, Barba JJ, Rodríguez NH. La importancia del aprendizaje reflexivo en el Practicum de Magisterio: una revisión de la literatura. Revista de Docencia Universitaria. 2015;**13**(3):147-170

[30] Ramsey C. Introducing Reflective Learning. Primera ed. Open University Worldwide: Thanet Press Limited; 2006

[31] Forneris S, Peden-Mcalpine C. Contextual learning: A reflective learning intervention for nursing education. International Journal of Nursing Education Scholarship. 2006;**3**(1):1-20

[32] Herrera Bastida EI, Durán Cárdenas C, Barona Nuñez AV. Investigación en educación interprofesional basada en simulación. Revista de la Facultad de Medicina de la Universidad Nacional Autónoma de México. 2019;**1**(1):1-14

[33] Rossit RAS, Dos Santos Junior CF, de Medeiros NMH, Medeiros LMOP, Regis CG, Batista SHSS. The research group as a learning scenario in/on interprofessional education: Focus on narratives. Interface: Communication, Health, Education. 2018;**22**(2):1511-1523

[34] Vergel J, Quintero GA, Forero Nieto SL, Espinosa AF, Aguia Rojas K, Quiroga Torres DA, et al. Módulos de educación interprofesional en la Escuela de Medicina y Ciencias de la Salud de la Universidad del Rosario. Bucaramanga, Colombia: Poster session presented at Tercer taller nacional de Educación Interprofesional; 2019

[35] Reeves S, Pelone F, Harrison R, Goldman J, Zwarenstein M. Interprofessional collaboration to improve professional practice and healthcare outcomes. Cochrane Database of Systematic Reviews. 2017;**6**(6):1-40

[36] Jiménez Martínez CA, Amato D, Duhart Hernández MG, Flores Mondragón MA, Gómez Clavel JF, Lara Barrón AM, et al. Teorías y creencias de universitarios respecto a los equipos interprofesionales de atención a la salud. Psicología Iztacala. 2019;**22**(4):2896-2917

Chapter 3

Resilience in the Future of Medical Education

Edie L. Sperling, Davis Mendel and Jennifer M. Hulett

Abstract

Personal resilience is known to decline during medical school without targeted intervention. While causal research remains limited, there is a clear correlation between diminished resilience and the heightened stress and anxiety that medical students often experience throughout their training. This chapter explores the various approaches that have been tested to address resilience among medical students, including curricular, extracurricular, preclinical, and clinical interventions, as well as those guided by mental health professionals. A critical examination of the concept of personal resilience is conducted, and personal resilience as a solution to the wider issues within healthcare that are influencing medical trainee burnout is challenged. Research on how Generation Z navigates the challenges of medical school is presented with the purpose of informing medical faculty and institutions for the future of medical education. Finally, sustainable and comprehensive strategies for fostering environments that support and strengthen resilience in medical students are proposed.

Keywords: resilience, stress, Gen Z, medical students, medical education

1. Introduction

It is well-known that high levels of stress and mental health concerns begin very early in medical school [1–3] and resilience declines over the course of training [4–6]. A third of medical students have positive screens for depression, and a quarter of medical students indicate increased mental health needs after starting medical school [7, 8]. Medical students have a rapid increase in suicidality and suicide attempts after beginning schooling [9, 10]. This trend may continue into professional life, with rates of depression, substance use disorder, suicide, burnout, job turnover, and complete occupational attrition higher in healthcare professionals than any other profession [11–13]. More than a third of healthcare professionals report an intent to leave healthcare within the next year [12, 13].

It is clear that physicians and medical students have mental health challenges [14, 15]. Though there have been a plethora of solutions proposed, attempts to increase personal resilience are some of the most commonly trialed [16–28]. The term "resilience" typically refers to personal resilience or the resilience of an individual and is defined as someone who thrives and adapts in spite of challenges, copes with stress successfully and in healthy ways, and does not give up after a failure [29]. Resilience is considered trainable in most conceptual models [29].

Personal resilience puts the burden on individuals to learn and employ new coping skills [30]. Responsibility or blame may fall on the individual if they do not prove "resilient enough" in managing stress [30]. Recent research has noted that placing the responsibility for resilience on individual physicians and medical students while there are clearly systemic issues within healthcare contributing to burnout [29] is likely ignoring the root of the problem [31].

Current research is scant on specific causes of personal resilience decline during medical school [4–6], although previous research demonstrates that resilience remains low throughout residency [32–34]. A rebound in resilience appears to occur in many physicians at some point after transitioning to professional practice, as physicians report higher resilience than the general U.S. population [35]. This chapter [1] explores what has been tried to assist with medical students' stress and personal resilience, [2] critically examines the concept of personal resilience as a solution for a healthcare system in crisis, [3] describes the current research on Generation Z (Gen Z) and hypothesizes about its meaning for Gen Z medical students, and [4] lists recommendations for creating environments which foster resilience among Gen Z medical students.

2. Methodology

A systematic review was conducted *via* the Preferred Reporting Items for Systematic Review and MetaAnalyses (PRISMA) guidelines to find all relevant literature on resilience training among medical students [36]. Inclusion criteria were: [1] describes an intervention designed to improve resilience, broadly inclusive of didactic education, cognitive techniques, group psychodynamics, and mindfulness training with the goal of increasing resilience; [2] medical student population including medical doctor (MD), doctor of osteopathy (DO), and international training programs; [3] primary studies of single-arm pre-post design, randomized controlled trial (RCT), or two-arm non-randomized studies; and [4] written in or translated into English. No restrictions were placed on study location or date.

The following databases were searched: EBSCOhost (inclusive of Academic Search Elite; Alt Healthwatch; Business Source Elite; CINAHL; eBook Collection; ERIC; Funk & Wagnalls New World Encyclopedia; Health Source – Consumer Edition; Health Source – Nursing/Academic Edition; Library, Information Science & Technology Abstracts; MAS Ultra – School Edition; Military & Government Collection; Newspaper Source; Primary Search; OpenDissertations; APA PsycINFO; MAS Reference eBook Collection; Primary Search Reference eBook Collection; and MEDLINE); EBSCO Discovery, in the categories Complementary & Alternative Medicine, Health & Medicine, Psychology, and Public Health; PubMed; Trip; Web of Science; Sociological Abstracts; SveMed+; Education Full Text; and Education Index Retrospective (available titles are between 1923 and 1983). Information was extracted and coded *via* a previously developed codebook [37]. The search terms included "resilience," "resiliency," and "medical students." Zotero and Excel were used for data management. See **Figure 1**.

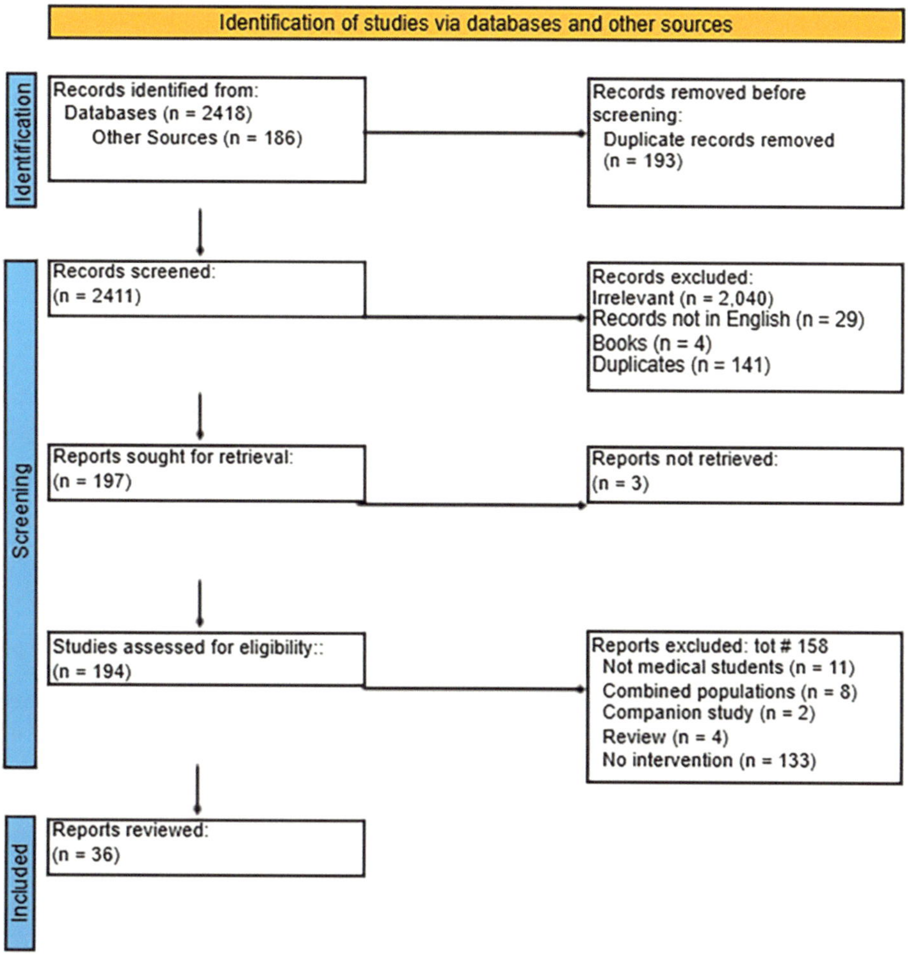

Figure 1.
PRISMA flowchart [36].

3. Resilience interventions among medical students

Many interventions to build personal resilience have been tested among medical students with mixed results [6, 20–23, 27, 38–50]. Numerous interventions at the time of this writing are in the feasibility stage, without data from randomized trials or control group comparisons [20, 22, 23, 27, 40–42, 44–49]. Even so, some interventions have resulted in significant improvements in resilience [6, 20, 21, 38, 39, 43], which is promising for further research. A brief review of the state of the science follows. See **Table 1** for a summary of all articles.

Multiple interventions have targeted preclinical medical students. Babal et al. [38] carried out an eight-week extracurricular intervention for $n = 32$ preclinical medical students with meal-sharing and the practice of resilience skills including perspective, empathy, and self-compassion [38]. Resilience significantly improved (0.4; CI, 0.2-0.5; $p < 0.01$) and the change was maintained up to the final measurement point, six months post-intervention [38]. Chan et al. [21] developed and delivered the

Study/Location	Design	Intervention	Sample Characteristics	Outcome measures*/Results
Babal et al. [38] United States	Single-arm pre-post	Extracurricular elective on perspective, empathy, self-compassion Duration: 8 weeks (3 cohorts) Total number of sessions: 8	N = 32, preclinical Age: 81.2% aged 20–24% female: 81.3	Outcome measures: BRS, IRI-PT/IRI-EC, Neff Self-Compassion Scale Results: Resilience significantly improved (0.4; CI, 0.2–0.5; $p < 0.01$)
Bird et al. [20] United States	Single-arm pre-post	Resilience workshops: reflection on stressors, managing setbacks, finding meaning Duration: unknown weeks; 1 hr. ea. Total number of sessions: 4	N = 144, clinical Mean age: not reported % female: not reported	Outcome measures: CD-RISC, acceptability Results: One cohort had significantly improved resilience ($MD = 2.7$, $p = 0.02$) and one did not
Brown et al. [39] United Kingdom	Single-arm pre-post	Stoic training (online) Duration: 15–20 mins per day x 12 days Total number of sessions: 12	N = 24, third-year Mean age: 21% female: 62.5	Outcome measures: BRS, SABS, JSE Results: Resilience increased significantly from pre- to post-training ($t(23) = 2.37$, $p = 0.02, d = 0.50$)
Bynum et al. [40] United States	Single-arm pre-post	A Resilience Seminar: Recognizing and Constructively Engaging with Shame Duration: 2 hours Total number of sessions: 1	N = 113 (62 completed outcome measure) Mean age: not reported % female: not reported	Outcome measures: self-developed survey Results: improved recognition of and attitude towards shame
Chan et al. [21] Australia	Single-arm pre-mid-post	MaRIS (Mindfulness, affective Reflection, Impactive experience, Supportive environment) Duration: 21 x 3 hours each Total number of sessions: 21	N = 55, first-year Age: 52.7% ≤21; 47.3% ≥22% female: 52.7	Outcome measures: self-developed MIQ Results: Resilience significantly improved ($t = 3.46, p = 0.001$)
Cheung et al. [41] United States	Single-arm pre-post	LAVENDER (Leveraging Affect and Valuing Empathy for Nurturing Doctors' Emotional Resilience) Duration: 30–45 mins each, monthly Total number of sessions: 4	N = 157, third-year/clinical Mean age: 25.88 ($SD = 2.25$) % female: 49	Outcome measures: PSS-4, MBI, acceptability Results: 76% of participants reported skills were useful; 72% would recommend; decreased positive emotion ($F = 4.09, p = 0.007$); increased burnout ($F = 3.61$, $p = 0.01$)

Study/Location	Design	Intervention	Sample Characteristics	Outcome measures*/Results
Dyrbye et al. [42] United States	Single-arm pre-post	SMART (Stress Management and Resilience Training) Duration: 1 academic year; 12 hrs (cohort 1)/10 hrs (cohort 2) Total number of sessions: 8	N = 48/47 (cohort 1/cohort 2), first-year/ preclinical Mean age: 77.1/79.5% ages <25% female: 58.3/59.1	Outcome measures: MBI, SF-8, PSS, CD-RISC-2, Happiness & Gratitude Scale Results: Quality-of-life decreased (cohort 1 $MD = -5.63, p < 0.001$ and cohort 2 $MD = -5.15$, $p = 0.02$); happiness decreased (cohort 1 $MD = -0.31, p = 0.02$ and cohort 2 $MD = -0.4$, $p = 0.01$); stress increased (cohort 1 $MD = 4.22, p = < 0.0001$ and cohort 2 $MD = 3.62$, $p = 0.03$); no resilience change
Edmonds et al. [43] United States	Single-arm pre-post	Wellness curriculum with mental health service, seminars, committee Duration: academic year Total number of sessions: dependent on student	N = 49, preclinical Age: 65.5% ages 24–29% female: 48.3	Outcome measures: WHO-5, PSS Results: overall wellbeing increased over the course of the year ($F(2,105) = 4.36$, $p = 0.015$)
Ekbäck et al. [22] Sweden	Single-arm pre-post	TARA (Training for Awareness, Resilience and Action) Duration: 12 weeks Total number of sessions: 12	N = 23 Mean age: 25.38% female: 78.2%	Outcome measures: Child Session Rating Scale, HADS, PSS-10, AFQ Results: feasible with a score of 34.99 out of 40.00; insignificant change other outcomes
Gheihman et al. [23] United States	Single-arm pre-post	Everyday Resilience Duration: 90 mins Total number of sessions: 1	N = 17 Mean age: not reported % female: not reported	Outcome measures: self-developed acceptability Results: 16 felt the workshop was 'valuable' or 'very valuable'
Jeyasingam [44] Australia	Single-arm post survey	Tutorials on philosophy of medicine, medical ethics, decision-making Duration: three x two hours each Total number of sessions: 3	N = 140, clinical Mean age: not reported % female: not reported	Outcome measures: self-developed acceptability Results: 70–80% of respondents agreed or strongly agreed with the statement "Information was relevant to me at my stage of training"

Study/Location	Design	Intervention	Sample Characteristics	Outcome measures*/Results
Kaligis et al. [45] Indonesia	RCT	Online mental-health strengthening modules Duration: 5 weeks, 45 mins per session Total number of sessions: 7	N = 105 (n = 52 intervention group/n = 53 control group) first-year Age: 59.62%/81.13% age 18% female: 53.85/67.92	Outcome measures: CD-RISC, PSS, DASS, TSST, salivary cortisol, alpha-amylase Results: no self-rated change in resilience; significant decrease in salivary cortisol in intervention group ($MD = -3.84, p < 0.001$)
Kempf & Hayton [46] United States	Single-arm post	Advanced Integration Weeks on compassion science, recognizing suffering, etc. Duration: not reported Total number of sessions: not reported	N = not reported; third-year/clinical Mean age: not reported % female: not reported	Outcome measures: not reported Results: 93% found value in sessions; 74% more confident in recognizing and acknowledging suffering in themselves and others; 83% rated compassion as critical to patient care
Kiesewetter & Dimke [47] Germany	Single-arm post	Emotional Speed-Dating guided with 6 questions about emotional experiences Duration: 3 mins x 4 rounds Total number of sessions: 1	N = not reported Mean age: not reported % female: not reported	Outcome measure: not reported Results: increased student empowerment to share emotions
Mugford et al. [27] United States	Single-arm post	ART (Active Resilience Training) Duration: not reported Total number of sessions: 5	N = 35 Mean age: not reported % female: not reported	Outcome measure: self-developed acceptability survey Results: 80% reported using skills learned at least weekly; 94% reported ART was somewhat, very, or extremely effective in teaching long-term useable skills
Sperling & Hudson [6]	Two-arm quasi-experimental	Small psychoeducational process group led by psychiatrist Duration: academic year Total number of sessions: 25	N = 16 (n = 8/8 intervention/ control groups) Mean age: 28.6/25.4% female: 75/63	Outcome measures: CD-RISC-25, PSS-10, Grit-O Results: resilience significantly decreased in the control group ($n = 8$, $t = -2.91, p = 0.03$); maintained in intervention group
Thomas et al. [49] United States	Single-arm post	Resilience extracurricular program: mental health, help-seeking, stress resilience Duration: 1 hr. sessions Total number of sessions: 7	N = not reported Mean age: not reported % female: not reported	Outcome measures: acceptability survey Results: 85% agreed presentations contained useful information; 41–88% found information useful for their future

Study/Location	Design	Intervention	Sample Characteristics	Outcome measures*/Results
Williams et al. [50] United States	Single-arm pre-post	PRIMe (Promoting Resilience in Medicine) elective Duration: 2 hours x 11 weeks Total number of sessions: 11	N = 24 Mean age: not reported % female: 70.8	Outcome measures: FMI, PSS, acceptability Results: FMI improved (M = 34.4 (6.10) to M = 41.8 (4.81), p not reported)

**Legend: AFQ: Avoidance and Fusion Questionnaire for youth; BRS: Brief Resilience Scale; CD-RISC: Connor-Davidson Resilience Scale (multiple versions); DASS: Depression Anxiety Stress Scale; FMI: Freiberg Mindfulness Inventory; Grit-O: Original Grit Scale; HADS: Hospital Anxiety and Depression Scale; IRI-PT/IRI-EC: Interpersonal Reactivity Index Perspective-Taking and Empathetic Concern scales; JES: Jefferson Empathy Scale; MBI: Maslach Burnout Inventory; MIQ: MARIs Impact Questionnaire; PSS: Perceived Stress Scale (multiple versions); SABS: Stoic Attitudes and Behavior Scale; SF-8: Medical Outcomes Study Short-Form-8; TSST: Trier Social Stress Test; WHO-5: World Health Organization Wellbeing Index.*

Table 1.
Resilience interventions for medical students: Literature summary.

MaRIS model (Mindfulness, affective Reflection, Impactive experience, Supportive environment) to n = 55 first-year students at Griffith University School of Medicine [21]. MaRIS focused on communication skills and constructive management of stress, including simulated clinical sessions with standardized patients, and resilience increased significantly (t = 3.46, p = 0.001) [21]. Edmonds et al. [43] at the Mayo Clinic Alix School of Medicine-AZ created a multifaceted “wellness curriculum” for preclinical students, including mental health services, curricular seminars, and a wellness committee of students, faculty, and staff, that offered programming, and student-led wellness activities [43]). It was found that of the n = 49 students who filled out the survey, students engaged most with student-initiated programming, which included intramural soccer, an improvisation class, an exercise equipment lending library, and a cooking class [43]). Resilience was not specifically measured, but overall well-being increased over the course of the year (F(2,105) = 4.36, p = 0.015) [43]).

Interventions have also targeted students on clinical rotations. Jeyasingam [44] piloted three, two-hour tutorials at Western Sydney University during the first year of clinical rotations on the philosophy of medicine, medical ethics, and medical decision-making for n = 140 students [44]. 70–80% of respondents agreed or strongly agreed with the statement “(This) information was relevant to me at my stage of training” [44]. Bird et al. [20] delivered four resilience workshops for n = 144 clinical students in which they reflected on stressors they were experiencing, including difficult team dynamics and uncertainty [20]. Training included letting go of negative emotions, how to manage setbacks, and finding meaning in day-to-day work [20]. Out of the two cohorts that went through the training, one significantly improved resilience (MD = 2.7, p = 0.02) and one did not [20]. A trial by Brown et al. [39] at Hull York Medical School delivered stoic training online for n = 24 third-year medical students over 12 days [39]. The stoic philosophy teaches how to process negative emotions while maintaining human connection, accepting things we cannot change, and taking ethical action [39]. Resilience increased significantly from pre- to post-training ($t(23)$ = 2.37, p = 0.02, d = 0.50) [39].

Several trials have noted a decrease in resilience or resilience-associated factors, or no change in resilience. LAVENDER (Leveraging Affect and Valuing Empathy for Nurturing Doctors' Emotional Resilience) was a program developed by Cheung et al. [41] at the Albert Einstein College of Medicine that aimed to increase positive emotion to preserve well-being in $n = 157$ third-year medical students [41]. 76% of participants reported the skills they learned in LAVENDER were useful, and 72% would recommend LAVENDER to others [41]. However, students reported decreased positive emotion ($F = 4.09, p = 0.007$) and increased burnout ($F = 3.61, p = 0.01$); there was no control group for comparison [41]. A required stress management and resilience course for first-year students developed by Dyrbye et al. [42] at the Mayo Clinic School of Medicine was based on the Stress Management and Resilience Training (SMART) program, focused on awareness, attention to the present moment, gratitude, compassion, and acceptance [42]. Quality-of-life (Cohort 1 $MD = -5.63$, $p < 0.001$ and Cohort 2 $MD = -5.15, p = 0.02$) and happiness scores (Cohort 1 $MD = -0.31, p = 0.02$ and Cohort 2 $MD = -0.4, p = 0.01$) declined significantly while stress increased (Cohort 1 $MD = 4.22, p = < 0.0001$ and Cohort 2 $MD = 3.62$, $p = 0.03$); there was no change in resilience in either cohort [42].

Feasibility studies have demonstrated that resilience training is feasible in medical school environments [6, 20–23, 27, 38–50]. Bynum et al. [40] delivered a shame resilience seminar for $n = 113$ ($n = 62$ complete pre/post survey responses) second-year medical students at Duke University, given in two hours in a large group/small group format [40]. Students demonstrated improved recognition of shame (for example, one of the survey questions asked "How confident are you in your ability to recognize when you are experiencing shame?") and attitude around shame (for example, "How comfortable would you feel sharing your feelings of shame with a peer?") immediately after the session [40]. Advanced Integration Weeks for third-year students were also rated as helpful in a study Loma Linda University School of Medicine by Kempf and Hayton [46], which included a week of lectures, practical training, community service, career development, and electives on compassion science and recognizing suffering in oneself and others [46]. An Emotional Speed-Dating intervention was delivered by Kiesewetter and Dimke [47] that involved pairs of students asking each other six questions in three minutes about emotions they saw in patients, which emotions were more or less difficult to manage for them, and which ones surprised them [47]. Students reported that the dialog helped normalize shared difficulties in dealing with patients' and their own emotions such as frustration and helplessness, with 74% more confident in recognizing and acknowledging suffering in themselves and others and 83% rating compassion as critical to patient care [47].

Training for Awareness, Resilience, and Action (TARA) was designed by Ekbäck et al. [22] to prevent depression, anxiety, stress, and burnout in first-year medical students at the Umeå University School of Medicine [22]. Breath work, slow movements, psychoeducation, interpersonal activities, and value-based committed action were introduced to $n = 23$ students in the 12-week program, which was found to be feasible with a score of 34.99 out of 40.00 on the Child Session Rating Scale [22]. At Harvard University, Gheihman et al. [23] produced a student-led 90-minute interactive workshop entitled Everyday Resilience, taught using two skills worksheets to encourage reflection on identifying one's strengths and thinking about resilience as a daily practice [23]. Of the $n = 17$ students who completed the workshop and pre/post measures, 16 felt the workshop was "valuable" or "very valuable" [23]. Active Resilience Training (ART) was developed by Mugford et al. [27] at Wake Forest School of Medicine and focused on teaching $n = 35$ students sleep prioritization, building support systems, mindfulness techniques, and planned breaks [27]. 80% of students reported using the skills what they had learned at least weekly, and 94%

reported that ART was somewhat, very, or extremely effective in teaching long-term useable skills [27]. In a study by Thomas et al. [49] at the Medical University of South Carolina, a pilot of a resilience extracurricular program included presentations on mental health, help-seeking, and stress resilience for first-year students [49]. 85% of the student who attended agreed that presentations contained useful information for maintaining balance during medical school; 41–88% considered the information useful for their future [49]. Developed by Williams et al. [50], Promoting Resilience in Medicine (PRIMe) was an eleven-week elective at the University of Florida College of Medicine that taught mindfulness and meditation skills and aimed to increase social support [50]. $N = 24$ students reported increased mindfulness ($MD = 7.4$, p not reported) with no change in stress ratings; resilience was not specifically measured [50].

Relatively few studies included objective measures, with the exception of Kaligis et al. [45] who delivered a four-week online intervention to $n = 52$ first-year students (control group $n = 53$) consisting of four weekly mental health-strengthening modules for medical students at Universitas Indonesia [45]. No significant change in resilience was found, but there was a significant decrease in salivary cortisol in the intervention group ($MD = -3.84$, $p < 0.001$) after 12 weeks [45].

Only four known studies have trialed interventions for medical students utilizing mental health professionals as facilitators [6, 26, 51, 52] and only one of these specifically targeted resilience [6]. In this pilot by Sperling and Hudson [6], resilience significantly decreased in the control group ($n = 8$, $t = -2.91$, $p = 0.03$) while not changing significantly from pre-intervention levels in the intervention group ($n = 8$) suggesting that interventions during medical school may not improve resilience so much as prevent its usual decline [6]. More research is needed to illuminate this issue.

4. The culture of medicine

Dr. Chris Watling noted: "Medicine's historical tendency to build stress-resistant individuals rather than to build wellness-supporting environments may reflect the values of the profession" [53]. The culture of medicine has long had a reputation for individuals who put others' needs before their own, eschew seeking help, and rarely take time off [53–55]. This paradigm has started to shift only within the past ten to fifteen years, likely due to a wider cultural shift acknowledging mental health challenges and advocating for reduced mental health stigma [56]. This shift gained momentum during the COVID-19 pandemic, but substantive change for healthcare professionals is still lacking [56]. Perceived problems within medicine and medical training that lead to burnout include both internal and external factors, for instance, a lack of autonomy [57] and the second-victim phenomenon [58], among others. Components of the culture of medicine that have been linked to resilience are described below.

4.1 The physician personality

Gabbard [54] coined the term "physician personality" when he identified a triad of common traits among many physicians: doubt, feelings of guilt, and an exaggerated sense of responsibility [54]. Maladaptive manifestations included inability to relax, resistance to using vacation time, poor boundaries, issues balancing work/home life, a chronic sense of "not doing enough," and poor self-care [54]. Recent research has supported that maladaptive behaviors may persist in the present day, noting that common physician qualities including attention to detail, perseverance, empathy, and service to others, which can convert into obsessiveness, perfectionism, and self-neglect when they experience high levels of stress [55].

The "Big 5" personality traits have been researched among medical students: extraversion, agreeableness, conscientiousness, openness, and neuroticism [59]. Individuals with higher neuroticism have an elevated stress response and thus are more susceptible to negative emotions [60]. Medical students with high extraversion and conscientiousness and low neuroticism have been found to have better clinical performance [59]. Medical students with higher stress levels have been found to have higher neuroticism as well as higher agreeableness [61], suggesting students with these personality traits may be more susceptible to stress.

However, personality is not created in a vacuum, nor is a dysregulated stress response [60]. Research supports that neuroticism has an environmental component [60]. A predisposition to view events negatively may be partially inherited vulnerability (e.g., amygdala excitability), partially due to childhood experiences of unpredictability and uncontrollability, and partially a learned behavior [60]. Placing the onus on medical students and physicians to adapt their so-called personality traits when their environment is highly stressful may be faulty logic. Medical students are placed in an environment with experienced physicians and mirroring their behaviors and responses—the very basis of clinical rotations and residency training [62]. When burnout is the norm, burnout could be a learned behavior.

4.2 Imposter syndrome

Imposter syndrome was first described by Clance and Imes in 1978 as an internal sense of being unintelligent despite evidence to the contrary [63]. Individuals felt they had fooled everyone who perceived them as intelligent or successful [63]. Imposter syndrome remains widespread today among highly successful individuals [64]. It can increase one's motivation to achieve, but it is also linked to high levels of emotional exhaustion, work–family conflict, anxiety, depression, guilt, job dissatisfaction, burnout, and suicidality [55, 64]. Medical student imposter syndrome prevalence is estimated between 20% and 60% with female-identifying individuals typically more impacted [64, 65]. High resilience may be protective against imposter syndrome among medical students [66].

However, institutional culture also plays a role in imposter syndrome [64]. For example, a culture that punishes mistakes may create a psychologically unsafe learning environment [64]. A medical school culture supportive of students, which accepts mistakes, and which is focused on growth over perfection may produce graduates with lower imposter syndrome and higher resilience.

4.3 Autonomy

Autonomy is the desire to organize one's own experiences and behaviors and to make one's own choices without the influence of outside pressures [67, 68]. The requirements of accreditation compounded with the time constraints of medical training can lead to significantly decreased personal choice during medical training; for example, students typically do not choose a major, minor, or pacing of coursework; electives are limited or nonexistent, and there is much less time for extracurricular activities [57]. Medical education may present a sudden reduction in choices for students compared to undergraduate schooling, making the transition to medical school even more difficult [57].

Most medical students are in the developmental stage of emerging adulthood, a period characterized by a desire for greater autonomy, and a lack of autonomy in this phase can hinder their natural growth and development [69]. Missing basic psychological needs fulfillment, including autonomy, has been shown to be related to higher stress among medical students [70]. Autonomy continues to be a point of contention among practicing physicians, who perceive lack of autonomy as a direct contributor to burnout and one of the top reasons they consider leaving clinical practice [71].

4.4 The second-victim phenomenon

Individuals who have witnessed traumatic events or their aftermath may develop sadness, guilt, anxiety, and/or signs and symptoms consistent with post-traumatic stress disorder, termed the "second-victim syndrome" [58, 72]. This is very common among healthcare professionals, who frequently engage with patients' trauma and pain [58, 72]. Supportive interventions directed at second victims have demonstrated success [58, 72], and individuals with higher resilience have been found to be better able to cope with being the second victim [73]. However, given that help-seeking is limited among healthcare professionals and students [74], and their time for personal care is decreased due to long work or studying hours [75], interventions may not be accessed.

Among healthcare students, common causes of the second victim phenomenon are witnessing or being involved with medication errors, patient falls, or errors during procedures [76]. In medical professionals, there are three possible outcomes in the theoretical model of the second victim: thriving, surviving, or leaving [76]. Among medical students there may only be two: giving up or moving on [76]. As support structures in institutions are directed at working professionals and not students, and medical schools may not have direct interventions designed for second victims, medical students may have less resources available for support after witnessing traumatic events [76]. While personal resilience may be protective for those with already high resilience [73], strategies and resources for those with less resilience—those whom have had less time or opportunity to develop personal resilience—are needed [76].

4.5 Challenges in the culture of medicine

An abundance of literature highlights a troubling reality about the culture that both physicians and medical students are immersed in [54, 55, 63–65, 74, 77, 78]. Physician culture often fosters a denial of personal health needs, particularly mental health [78, 79]. Factors such as imposter syndrome, lack of autonomy, and the second-victim phenomenon exacerbate the challenges of a profession and training system that contribute to burnout [64, 71, 74]. In addition, external pressures—such as climate change, inflation, high housing costs, and medical school debt—further deepen medical students' sense of uncertainty and loss of control over their futures [80–82].

5. Generation Z medical students

Gen Z includes individuals born between approximately 1995 and 2012 [83], making them between about 13 to 30 years old. In 2024, approximately 57% of U.S. medical school matriculants were between the ages of 23 and 25, and 26% were between the ages of 20 and 22 [84], meaning by 2030, medical school cohorts will primarily comprise Gen Z individuals.

Research supports that Gen Z individuals want to be involved in decision-making and are resistant to standard procedure; they want transparency, flexibility, personalized attention, and communication from leadership [85]. Gen Z individuals are likely to be efficient problem-solvers and "out of the box" thinkers [85]. These qualities may result in medical students that want to know the "why" behind curricular choices and feel their input should be respected and addressed by leadership. Gen Z students expect diversity to be an institutional priority and for practices to be corrected quickly that do not follow the principles of diversity, equity, and inclusion (DEI) [85]. For medical school lagging in incorporating DEI training and practices, Gen Z students may attempt to accelerate change.

Arnett's theory of emerging adulthood describes a delayed entry into adult roles that has become typical in Western society over the past several decades [69, 86]. Emerging adulthood describes a developmental stage between the ages of 18 to 29 [69], thus encompassing most medical students. Individuals in this approximate age range have been found to be less likely to exhibit the choices and behaviors than those in prior generations did at this age [69]. For example, emerging adults are less likely to have a long-term career and instead have temporary or part-time employment or be a student; are less likely to have a stable long-term relationship and instead are casually dating; and are less likely to be living independently and instead live with their parents [69]. Inflation and housing costs have contributed to these characteristics recently, making what may have initially been a choice a necessity [69].

Emerging adults are exploring their identities and what commitments they might want to make regarding career, relationships, and personal values; they value their freedom and are finding ways to exert their independence, a developmental phase that used to be primarily observed in adolescence [69]. While uncertainty and some degree of anxiety is normal during this stage, emerging adults currently have the highest incidence of depression, anxiety, and substance use disorder out of any age group [69], which may translate into the increasing stress, depression, and anxiety seen among medical students [1–3].

The loss of independence and flexibility experienced during medical school may contribute to an increased risk of mental health challenges and undermine resilience. Medical students who are uncertain of their career choice may be especially vulnerable as they navigate significant uncertainty in multiple aspects of their lives [69]. Medical training is both a lengthy (7 to 11 years; [87]) and costly ($160,000 to $320,000 not including interest for four years of medical school; [88]) endeavor, which makes the decision to persist in the face of doubts even more consequential than in many other career paths.

6. The fallacy of personal resilience

There have been many attempts to increase personal resilience among medical students [18–28, 31, 89]. However, there is limited research on changing environments to be more supportive – likely due to the many barriers to attempting organizational and systemic change within healthcare [90]. Two studies included elements of environmental change, including the MaRIS model, which used mentorship to reduce the anxiety and stress incited by learning new skills [21], and the Mayo Clinic Alix School of Medicine-AZ, which created a multifaceted "wellness curriculum"

[43]. Even in those cases, however, the onus was on the students to opt in and attend wellness activities [43].

Personal resilience puts the burden on individuals to learn and employ new coping skills [30]. Placing the responsibility for resilience on individual physicians and medical students while there are clearly systemic issues within healthcare contributing to burnout [91] is likely ignoring the causes of the issues [30]. In contrast, student suggestions for stress reduction generally focus on reducing sources of stress, not on boosting their own coping strategies [92]. Medical students emphasize that modifying stressful curricular elements including redistributing workload to be more uniform, prioritizing clinically relevant content, and moving to a pass/fail grading system would be beneficial to them [92].

Abolishing stress altogether would be unlikely to be beneficial, even if it were possible, as medical students are going into a stressful profession and developing stress-management skills and personal resilience prior to entering the workforce is essential [53, 92]. However, it seems clear that U.S. medical curricula is not fostering resilience and stress management in most cases [1–6]. The increased stress that students experience upon entering medical school does not qualify as training students to manage stress.

While personal resilience rebounds at some point once out of training and in professional practice [35], physicians still have higher rates of burnout, depression, substance use disorder, suicide, job turnover, and occupational attrition than any other profession [11–13], indicating that personal resilience is not the whole story. Curricular, organizational, institutional, cultural, and interpersonal factors must all be examined for their roles in burnout, and flexibility of healthcare systems for interventions that truly seek to change the status quo is vitally important.

7. Creating environments which foster resilience

Burnout is a workplace phenomenon characterized by feeling emotionally drained, disconnected, depersonalized, and unengaged [93]. "Workplace" is a general term applied to work of any kind; students' "workplace" is their school, and their "job" is academics [94]. Burnout measures may fail to capture the associated physical and social effects that a person in burnout experiences, resulting in solutions that fail to address physical, social, or spiritual factors along with emotional and psychological ones [77]. For example, medicine is the only profession in which work-life balance worsens with more education [77], leaving physicians with little time for activities that enhance bodily health, social connection, or spiritual needs. Personal resilience is important and assists up to a point, but coping skills require time to utilize them, and stress management requires time to de-stress.

Physician burnout has been found to be largely driven by organizational factors as opposed to personal ones, including excessive documentation requirements, insurance restrictions, long hours, overnight work, high patient load, short patient appointments, understaffing, and lack of autonomy [77, 91]. Medical student stress and burnout is also largely driven by organizational factors, including high academic workload, high-stakes exams, lack of free time, flexibility, and autonomy, and presenteeism [56, 95].

To counteract the conditions that are contributing to stress as well as building personal resilience to manage stress, we recommend the following steps for medical institutions, with a focus on Gen Z medical student needs [56, 95]:

1. Training and feedback for PhD and other non-clinician instructors on what content is clinically or board relevant, with a strong emphasis on "need-to-know" information.

2. Limited seat time so that students have flexible time for studying, resting, and pursuing their own interests.

3. Elective courses so students have increased autonomy over what they learn. Allowing students to vote on the electives offered might increase autonomy further.

4. A specified number of "mental health days" without needing an approved time-off request.

5. Grading of Pass/No Pass.

6. Stress management offerings at convenient times, guided by student suggestions and led by students.

7. Institutional support of student-lead activities and initiatives that foster connection and support.

8. On-demand stress management training for implementation immediately after a failure or setback.

9. Psychoeducation built into the curriculum from the beginning of the first year, including resilience principles such as growth mindset.

8. Conclusions

The landscape of medicine is undergoing profound transformation as we approach the 2030s, and medical training must evolve to meet these new realities. While personal resilience will be essential in navigating these challenges, it will not be sufficient on its own. Systemic change is urgently needed across the entire healthcare landscape. To thrive, medical students must be equipped with the skills to not only survive but also excel in an increasingly complex environment. It is crucial to identify and implement systemic interventions that foster supportive, sustainable environments for both medical students and healthcare professionals, ensuring that the next generation of clinicians is prepared to meet the demands of the future.

Acknowledgements

The authors thank the Western University of Health Sciences for the support supplied during the creation of this content and for implementing many of the suggestions above. No funding was received in the preparation of this chapter.

Conflict of interest

The authors declare no conflict of interest.

Author details

Edie L. Sperling[1*], Davis Mendel[1] and Jennifer M. Hulett[2]

1 Western University of Health Sciences, Lebanon, Oregon, USA

2 University of Missouri, Columbia, Missouri, USA

*Address all correspondence to: esperling@westernu.edu

References

[1] Brooks SK, Gerada C, Chalder T. Review of literature on the mental health of doctors: Are specialist services needed? Journal of Mental Health. 2011;**20**(2):146-156

[2] Hill MR, Goicochea S, Merlo LJ. In their own words: Stressors facing medical students in the millennial generation. Medical Education Online. 2018;**23**(1):1530558

[3] Kalmoe MC, Chapman MB, Gold JA, Giedinghagen AM. Physician suicide: A call to action. Missouri Medicine. 2019;**116**(3):211-216

[4] Jordan RK, Shah SS, Desai H, Tripi J, Mitchell A, Worth RG. Variation of stress levels, burnout, and resilience throughout the academic year in first-year medical students. PLoS One. 2020;**15**(10):e0240667. Available from: http://www.ncbi.nlm.nih.gov/pmc/articles/PMC7561113/

[5] Luibl L, Traversari J, Paulsen F, Scholz M, Burger P. Resilience and sense of coherence in first year medical students - a cross-sectional study. BMC Medical Education. 2021;**21**(142):1-10. Available from: https://www.ncbi.nlm.nih.gov/pmc/articles/PMC7934430/

[6] Sperling EL, Hudson MG. Examining the effects of a small process group on grit, resilience, and stress levels among medical students: A pilot study. The Journal for Specialists in Group Work. 2024;**49**(2-3):120-138

[7] Mazurkiewicz R, Korenstein D, Fallar R, Ripp J. The prevalence and correlations of medical student burnout in the pre-clinical years: A cross-sectional study. Psychology, Health & Medicine. 2012;**17**(2):188-195

[8] Rosiek A, Rosiek-Kryszewska A, Leksowski Ł, Leksowski K. Chronic stress and suicidal thinking among medical students. IJERPH. 2016;**13**(2):212

[9] Marcon G, Massaro Carneiro Monteiro G, Ballester P, Cassidy RM, Zimerman A, Brunoni AR, et al. Who attempts suicide among medical students? Acta Psychiatrica Scandinavica. 2020;**141**(3):254-264

[10] Seo C, Di Carlo C, Dong SX, Fournier K, Haykal KA. Risk factors for suicidal ideation and suicide attempt among medical students: A meta-analysis. PLoS One. 2021;**16**(12):e0261785

[11] Mohanty A, Kabi A, Mohanty A. Health problems in healthcare workers: A review. Journal of Family Medicine and Primary Care. 2019;**8**(8):2568

[12] Bryant-Genevier J, Rao CY, Lopes-Cardozo B, Kone A, Rose C, Thomas I, et al. Symptoms of depression, anxiety, post-traumatic stress disorder, and suicidal ideation among state, tribal, local, and territorial public health workers during the COVID-19 pandemic—United States, march–April 2021. MMWR. Morbidity and Mortality Weekly Report. 2021;**70**(26):947-952

[13] Windover AK, Martinez K, Mercer MB, Neuendorf K, Boissy A, Rothberg MB. Correlates and outcomes of physician burnout within a large academic medical center. JAMA Internal Medicine. 2018;**178**(6):856

[14] de Cordova PB, Johansen ML, Grafova IB, Crincoli S, Prado J, Pogorzelska-Maziarz M. Burnout and intent to leave during COVID-19: A

cross-sectional study of New Jersey hospital nurses. Journal of Nursing Management. 2022;**30**(6):1913-1921

[15] Rotenstein LS, Brown R, Sinsky C, Linzer M. The association of work overload with burnout and intent to leave the job across the healthcare workforce during COVID-19. Journal of General Internal Medicine. 2023;**38**:1920-1927

[16] Shanafelt TD, Boone S, Tan L, Dyrbye LN, Sotile W, Satele D, et al. Burnout and satisfaction with work-life balance among US physicians relative to the general US population. Archives of Internal Medicine. 2012;**172**(18):1377

[17] Dyrbye LN, West CP, Satele D, Boone S, Tan L, Sloan J, et al. Burnout among U.S. medical students, residents, and early career physicians relative to the general U.S. population. Academic Medicine. 2014;**89**(3):443-451

[18] Angelopoulou P, Panagopoulou E. Resilience interventions in physicians: A systematic review and meta-analysis. Applied Psychology: Health and Well Being. 2022;**14**(1):3-25

[19] Bano Z, Pervaiz S. The relationship between resilience, emotional intelligence and their influence on psychological wellbeing: A study with medical students. Pakistan Armed Forces Medical Journal. 2020;**70**(2):390-394

[20] Bird A, Tomescu O, Oyola S, Houpy J, Anderson I, Pincavage A. A curriculum to teach resilience skills to medical students during clinical training. MedEdPORTAL. 2020:10975

[21] Chan K, Humphreys L, Mey A, Holland C, Wu C, Rogers G. Beyond communication training: The MaRIS model for developing medical students' human capabilities and personal resilience. Medical Teacher. 2020;**42**(2):187-195. Available from: http://pubmed.ncbi.nlm.nih.gov/31608726/

[22] Ekbäck E, Von Knorring J, Burström A, Hunhammar D, Dennhag I, Molin J, et al. Training for awareness, resilience and action (TARA) for medical students: A single-arm mixed methods feasibility study to evaluate TARA as an indicated intervention to prevent mental disorders and stress-related symptoms. BMC Medical Education. 2022;**22**(1):132

[23] Gheihman G, Cooper C, Simpkin A. Everyday resilience: Practical tools to promote resilience among medical students. Journal of General Internal Medicine. 2019;**34**(4):498-501

[24] Healy C, Ryan Á, Moran CN, Harkin DW, Doyle F, Hickey A. Medical students, mental health and the role of resilience—A cross-sectional study. Medical Teacher. 2023;**45**(1):40-48

[25] Lack L, Yielder J, Goodyear-Smith F. Evaluation of a compulsory reflective group for medical students. Journal of Primary Health Care. 2019;**11**(3):227

[26] Melo-Carrillo A, Van Oudenhove L, Lopez-Avila A. Depressive symptoms among Mexican medical students: High prevalence and the effect of a group psychoeducation intervention. Journal of Affective Disorders. 2012;**136**(3):1098-1103

[27] Mugford H, O'Connor C, Danelson K, Popoli D. Medical students' perceptions and retention of skills from active resilience training. Family Medicine. 2022;**54**(3):213-215

[28] Nair B, Otaki F, Nair AF, Ho SB. Medical students' perception of resilience and of an innovative curriculum-based resilience skills building course: A

participant-focused qualitative analysis. PLoS One. 2023;**18**(3):e0280417

[29] Connor KM, Davidson JRT. Development of a new resilience scale: The Connor-Davidson resilience scale (CD-RISC). Depression and Anxiety. 2003;**18**:76-82

[30] Cunningham T. Viewpoint: The burden of resilience should not fall solely on nurses. American Journal of Nursing. 2020;**120**(9):11

[31] Solomonian L, Crawford L, Mohmand S, Monteiro S, Neves T. Supporting medical student wellness during a pandemic: A pilot study of an extra-curricular resilience-promotion program. The CAND Journal. 2023;**30**(2):4-13

[32] Bird AN, Pincavage AT. Initial characterization of internal medicine resident resilience and association with stress and burnout. Journal of Biomedical Education. 2016;**2016**(1):3508638

[33] Nituica C, Bota OA, Blebea J, Cheng CI, Slotman GJ. Factors influencing resilience and burnout among resident physicians—A National Survey. BMC Medical Education. 2021;**21**(1):514

[34] Nituica C, Bota OA, Blebea J. Specialty differences in resident resilience and burnout—A national survey. The American Journal of Surgery. 2021;**222**(2):319-328

[35] West CP, Dyrbye LN, Sinsky C, Trockel M, Tutty M, Nedelec L, et al. Resilience and burnout among physicians and the general US working population. JAMA Network Open. 2020;**3**(7):e209385

[36] Page MJ, McKenzie JE, Bossuyt PM, Boutron I, Hoffmann TC, Mulrow CD, et al. The PRISMA 2020 statement: An updated guideline for reporting systematic reviews. BMJ. 2021;**372**(71):1-9. DOI: 10.1136/bmj.n71

[37] Cooper H. Research Synthesis and Meta-Analysis: A Step-by-Step Approach. 5th ed. Thousand Oaks, CA: Sage Publications, Inc.; 2017

[38] Babal JC, Eskola L, Jones A, Schultz RJ, Eickhoff JC. Medical student well-being outcomes after a novel shared meal and resiliency skills course. WMJ. 2023;**122**(4):272-276

[39] Brown MEL, MacLellan A, Laughey W, Omer U, Himmi G, LeBon T, et al. Can stoic training develop medical student empathy and resilience? A mixed-methods study. BMC Medical Education. 2022;**22**(1):340

[40] Bynum WE, Uijtdehaage S, Artino AR, Fox JW. The psychology of shame: A resilience seminar for medical students. MedEdPORTAL. 2020;**16**:11052

[41] Cheung EO, Kwok I, Ludwig AB, Burton W, Wang X, Basti N, et al. Development of a positive psychology program (LAVENDER) for preserving medical student well-being: A single-arm pilot study. Global Advances in Integrative Medicine and Health. 2021;**10**:2164956120988481

[42] Dyrbye L, Shanafelt T, Werner L, Sood A, Satele D, Wolanskyj A. The impact of a required longitudinal stress management and resilience training course for first-year medical students. Journal of General Internal Medicine. 2017;**32**(12):1309-1314. Available from: http://pubmed.ncbi.nlm.nih.gov/28861707/

[43] Edmonds VS, Chatterjee K, Girardo ME, Butterfield RJ III, Stonnington CM. Evaluation of a novel wellness curriculum on medical student

wellbeing and engagement demonstrates a need for student-driven wellness programming. Teaching and Learning in Medicine. 2022;**35**(1):52-64

[44] Jeyasingam N. Philosophy for resilience: A meaningful intervention for medical students. Journal of Academic Ethics. 2022;**20**(1):67-72

[45] Kaligis F, Ismail RI, Wiguna T, Prasetyo S, Gunardi H, Indriatmi W, et al. Effectiveness of an online mental health strengthening module to build resilience and overcome stress for transitional aged medical students. Frontiers in Digital Health. 2023;**5**:1207583

[46] Kempf H, Hayton A. Integration weeks: A novel way to build resilience in third year medical students. Medical Education. 2022;**56**(5):562

[47] Kiesewetter J, Dimke B. Emotional speed-dating as a part of medical students' resilience training. Medical Education. 2020;**54**(5):473-474

[48] Kulman-Lipsey S, Yang S, Pedram Javidan A, Fung B, Levinson A, Vernon J, et al. An integrative longitudinal resilience curriculum. The Clinical Teacher. 2019;**16**(4):395-400

[49] Thomas SE, Haney MK, Pelic CM, Shaw D, Wong JG. Developing a program to promote stress resilience and self-care in first-year medical students. Canadian Medical Education Journal. 2011;**2**(1):e32-e36

[50] Williams M, Estores I, Merlo L. Promoting resilience in medicine: The effects of a mind-body medicine elective to improve medical student well-being. Global Advances in Health and Medicine. 2020;**9**. Available from: http://pubmed.ncbi.nlm.nih.gov/32499968/ [Online]

[51] Liang L, Feng L, Zheng X, Wu Y, Zhang C, Li J. Effect of dialectical behavior group therapy on the anxiety and depression of medical students under the normalization of epidemic prevention and control for the COVID-19 epidemic: A randomized study. Annals of Palliative Medicine. 2021;**10**(10):10591-10599

[52] Samantaray NN, Nath B, Behera N, Mishra A, Singh P, Sudhir P. Brief cognitive behavior group therapy for social anxiety among medical students: A randomized placebo-controlled trial. Asian Journal of Psychiatry. 2021;**55**:102526

[53] Watling C. Tackling medical student stress: Beyond individual resilience. Perspectives on Medical Education. 2015;**4**(3):105-106

[54] Gabbard GO. The role of compulsiveness in the normal physician. JAMA. 1985;**254**(20):2926-2929

[55] Epstein RM, Privitera MR. Addressing physician mental health. The Lancet Psychiatry. 2019;**6**(3):190-191

[56] Lawler McHugh T, Fraone JS, Zhang Z. Mental health in the post-pandemic workplace: A culture shift towards transparency & empathy. Boston College Center for Work and Family; 2021. Available from: https://archive.hshsl.umaryland.edu/handle/10713/17351 [Online]

[57] Kusurkar RA, Croiset G. Autonomy support for autonomous motivation in medical education. Medical Education Online. 2015;**20**(1). Available from: https://pubmed.ncbi.nlm.nih.gov/25953033/ [Online]

[58] Nydoo PBJ, Naicker T, Moodley J. The second victim phenomenon in health care: A literature review. Scandanavian

Journal of Public Health. 2019;**48**(6):629-637. DOI: 10.1177/1403494819855506

[59] Peters H, Garbe A, Breil SM, Oberst S, Selch S, Holzhausen Y. Big five personality traits of medical students and workplace performance in the final clerkship year using an EPA framework. BMC Medical Education. 2024;**24**(1):453

[60] Barlow DH, Ellard KK, Sauer-Zavala S, Bullis JR, Carl JR. The origins of neuroticism. Perspectives on Psychological Science. 2014;**9**(5):481-496

[61] Le Saux O, Canada B, Debarnot U, Haouhache NEH, Lehot JJ, Binay M, et al. Association of personality traits with the efficacy of stress management interventions for medical students taking objective structured clinical examinations. Academic Medicine. 2024;**99**(7):784-793

[62] Raj KS. Well-being in residency: A systematic review. Journal of Graduate Medical Education. 2016;**8**(5):674-684

[63] Clance PR, Imes SA. The imposter phenomenon in high achieving women: Dynamics and therapeutic intervention. Psychotherapy: Theory, Research & Practice. 1978;**15**(3):241-247

[64] Gottlieb M, Chung A, Battaglioli N, Sebok-Syer SS, Kalantari A. Impostor syndrome among physicians and physicians in training: A scoping review. Medical Education. 2020;**54**(2):116-124

[65] Bagby-Stone S. Creating space for well-being in medical school and beyond. Missouri Medicine. 2021;**118**(1):50-54

[66] Camara GF, de Santiago Campos IF, Carneiro AG, de Sena Silva IN, de Barros Silva PG, Peixoto RAC, et al. Relationship between resilience and the impostor phenomenon among undergraduate medical students. Journal of Medical Education and Curricular Development. 2022;**9**:23821205221096105

[67] Cate OTJ t, Kusurkar RA, Williams GC. How self-determination theory can assist our understanding of the teaching and learning processes in medical education. AMEE guide No. 59. Medical Teacher. 2012;**33**(12):961-973

[68] Deci EL, Ryan RM. The "what" and "why" of goal pursuits: Human needs and the self-determination of behavior. Psychological Inquiry. 2000;**11**(4):227-268

[69] Arnett JJ, Žukauskienė R, Sugimura K. The new life stage of emerging adulthood at ages 18-29 years: Implications for mental health. The Lancet Psychiatry. 2014;**1**(7):569-576

[70] Neufeld A, Mossière A, Malin G. Basic psychological needs, more than mindfulness and resilience, relate to medical student stress: A case for shifting the focus of wellness curricula. Medical Teacher. 2020;**42**(12):1401-1412. DOI: 10.1080/0142159X.2020.1813876

[71] Melnikow J, Padovani A, Miller M. Frontline physician burnout during the COVID-19 pandemic: National survey findings. BMC Health Services Research. 2022;**22**(1):365

[72] Scott SD, Hirschinger LE, Cox KR, McCoig M, Brandt J, Hall LW. The natural history of recovery for the healthcare provider "second victim" after adverse patient events. Quality & Safety in Health Care. 2009;**18**(5):325-330

[73] Hernandez C. The role of resilience on second-victim outcomes: Examining individual and external factors of medical professionals [electronic theses and dissertations]. 6503; 2019. Available from: https://stars.library.ucf.edu/etd/6503

[74] Mehta SS, Edwards ML. Suffering in silence: Mental health stigma and physicians' licensing fears. American Journal of Psychiatry Residents' Journal. 2018;**13**(11):2-4

[75] Ray ME, Coon JM, Al-Jumaili AA, Fullerton M. Quantitative and qualitative factors associated with social isolation among graduate and professional health science students. AJPE. 2019;**83**(7):6983

[76] Catalán L, Alvarado-Peña J, Torres-Soto G, Lorca-Sepúlveda B, Besoain-Cornejo AM, Kappes M. Second victim phenomenon among healthcare students: A scoping review. Nurse Education in Practice. 2024;**79**:104094

[77] Abid R, Salzman G. Evaluating physician burnout and the need for organizational support. Missouri Medicine. 2021;**118**(3):185

[78] Gold JA, Johnson B, Leydon G, Rohrbaugh RM, Wilkins KM. Mental health self-care in medical students: A comprehensive look at help-seeking. Academic Psychiatry. 2015;**39**(1):37-46

[79] Davidson SK, Schattner PL. Doctors' health-seeking behaviour: A questionnaire survey. Medical Journal of Australia. 2003;**179**(6):302-305

[80] Dikeç G, Öztürk S, Taşbaşı N, Figenergül D, Güler BB. The perceptions of generation Z university students about their futures: A qualitative study. Sci. 2023;**5**(4):45

[81] Oladele OP, Uthman TJ, Babatunde SI, Aborisade TE. Exploring the relationship between economic hardship and suicidal ideation among gen Z and millennials: A comparative study. Ife Social Sciences Review. 2024;**32**(2):79-93

[82] Pisaniello MS, Asahina AT, Bacchi S, Wagner M, Perry SW, Wong ML, et al. Effect of medical student debt on mental health, academic performance and specialty choice: A systematic review. BMJ Open. 2019;**9**(7):e029980

[83] Eckleberry-Hunt J, Lick D, Hunt R. Is medical education ready for generation Z? Journal of Graduate Medical Education. 2018;**10**(4):378-381

[84] Association of American Medical Colleges. Matriculating Student Questionnaire (MSQ). (2024 All Schools Summary Report). 2024. Available from: https://www.aamc.org/media/64226/download

[85] Racolța-Paina ND, Irini RD. Quality-access to success. General Management. 2021;**22**(183):78-85

[86] Arnett JJ. Emerging Adulthood: The Winding Road from the Late Teens through the Twenties. Oxford, UK: Oxford University Press; 2004. 282 p

[87] Washington University School of Medicine in St. Louis. Residency Roadmap. Length of Residencies. 2025. Available from: https://residency.wustl.edu/residencies/length-of-residencies/

[88] The Princeton Review. How Much is Medical School? The Price of the White Coat | The Princeton Review. Available from: https://www.princetonreview.com/med-school-advice/how-much-is-medical-school

[89] Peng L, Li M, Zuo X, Miao Y, Chen L, Yu Y, et al. Application of the Pennsylvania resilience training program on medical students. Personality and Individual Differences. 2014;**61-62**:47-51

[90] "Siva" VS. Organizational change management in HealthCare. In: Johnson SM, Qureshi AP, Schlussel AT, Renton D, Jones DB, editors. The

SAGES Manual of Strategy and Leadership. Cham: Springer Nature Switzerland; 2024. pp. 511-533. DOI: 10.1007/978-3-031-62359-2_36

[91] Almutairi SF. Burnout among healthcare professionals: A review of causes, impacts, and alleviation strategies. Review of Contemporary Philosophy. 2023;**22**:43-52

[92] Kötter T, Pohontsch NJ, Voltmer E. Stressors and starting points for health-promoting interventions in medical school from the students' perspective: A qualitative study. Perspectives on Medical Education. 2015;**4**(3):128-135

[93] Maslach C, Goldberg J. Prevention of burnout: New perspectives. Applied & Preventive Psychology. 1998;7:63-74

[94] Kilic R, Nasello JA, Melchior V, Triffaux JM. Academic burnout among medical students: Respective importance of risk and protective factors. Public Health. 2021;**198**:187-195

[95] Fares J, Al Tabosh H, Saadeddin Z, El Mouhayyar C, Aridi H. Stress, burnout and coping strategies in preclinical medical students. North American Journal of Medicine and Science. 2016;**8**(2):75

Chapter 4

Usefulness of Attitude, Ethics, and Communication (AETCOM) Module of Competency-Based Medical Education

Abirlal Sen, Manidipa Barman and Sarjubala Thingujam

Abstract

The Attitude, Ethics, and Communication (AETCOM) module was introduced in 2019 to impart soft skills for the personal and professional development of medical students. AETCOM Module 1.3 deals with "Doctor-Patient relationship" which forms an integral part of clinical practice. This study was conducted to record reflections of first-year MBBS students regarding usefulness of AETCOM module 1.3. It was Mixed-method explorative study conducted in Department of Physiology, Tripura Medical College & Dr. BRAM Teaching Hospital upon first professional MBBS students. The Universal Sampling method was used. A Feedback questionnaire of eight questions was distributed and filled out by students at the end of AETCOM module 1.3. Responses were graded on a five-point Likert scale. Mean attitude score was generated. The result was expressed in terms of frequency, percentage, mean, and SD. As the maximum point of the Likert scale allotted to each question was 5, the overall attitude score of 8 questions is $5*8 = 40$. Out of 40, 71% of students had an attitude score > 35, while 29% of students had a score ≤ 35. 95% of Students agreed that AETCOM 1.3 helped them learn better. We concluded that teaching-learning of AETCOM module 1.3 can be an effective way for students to develop communication skills and doctor-patient relationships and to understand the professional qualities and roles of a physician.

Keywords: medical students, CBME, physiology, AETCOM, medical education, doctor-patient relationship

1. Introduction

The Attitude, Ethics, and Communication (AETCOM) module was introduced by the erstwhile Medical Council of India (MCI) in the Competency-Based Medical Education (CBME) curriculum in the year 2019, to impart soft skills for the personal and professional development of medical students. Among them, module 1.2 and

Module 1.3 have been assigned to the Physiology Department under the Competency-Based Medical Education (CBME) curriculum latest update dated 12 September 2024 [1]. Module 1.3 deals with "Doctor-Patient relationship" which forms an integral part of clinical practice.

An "Indian Medical Graduate" (IMG) should have knowledge, skills, attitudes, values, and alertness to function aptly as a physician of society and also be globally relevant [2]. This training module is a longitudinal program spread across all phases of the undergraduate medical program [3]. In the present study, we conducted a preliminary survey during the first phase of the competency program to find out students' reflection on the usefulness of AETCOM module 1.3 to develop their attitude, ethics, and communication skills toward patients.

2. Materials and method

The present study was conducted in the Department of Physiology, Tripura Medical College, and Dr. BRAM Teaching Hospital. It was a mixed-method explorative study. The sampling technique used was Universal sampling. The study duration was 6 months. Students of the first professional MBBS took part in the study.

2.1 Inclusion and exclusion criteria

Out of all students in Phase 1 MBBS of Batch 2024–2025, students who did not attend all the sessions of AETCOM module 1.3 and were not willing to participate in the study were excluded. Thus, a total of 87 students took part in the study.

2.2 Operational definitions

2.2.1 AETCOM module 1.3

AETCOM module 1.3 deals with the topic Doctor-Patient relationship, which forms an important part of clinical practice. AETCOM module 1.3 sessions were conducted by faculties of Dept. of Physiology, Tripura Medical College after completion of AETCOM module 1.2 sessions, which deals with the topic "What it means to be a patient?" as per NMC AETCOM module guidelines set for Physiology Undergraduate curriculum [4].

2.2.2 Conduct of sessions

AETCOM module 1.3 had four sessions, covering 7 hours viz.:

- Large group session – 1 hour
- Self-directed learning – 2 hours
- Interactive discussions – 2 hours
- Discussion and closure – 2 hours

AETCOM 1.3 Module addressed the following competencies:

- Enumerate and describe the professional qualities and roles of a physician
- Demonstrate empathy in patient encounters

2.2.3 Study tools

Reflective Notes: Opinions of the first professional MBBS students about the usefulness of the AETCOM module 1.3 were collected from the students through some reflective notes at the end of the AETCOM module 1.3 class (**Table 1**).

2.3 Data collection technique

- The procedure of the study was explained to the students and informed consent was taken from each student.
- The reflective notes from students were gathered through 8 close-ended questionnaires (viz. *real life situation, helped learning better, relevance, easy learning, can improve participation, helps gain competencies, enjoyable, preference for more AETCOM*), which was validated by IEC(H), Tripura Medical College and was distributed and filled by students at the end of AETCOM module 1.3.
- The feedback notes from students with assessment scores were analyzed statistically.
- Points were awarded for each question. All responses to the questions were categorized and graded on a Likert scale where 1 = Strongly Disagree, 2 = Disagree, 3 = Neutral, 4 = Agree, and 5 = Strongly Agree [5].
- Total score was calculated out of 40 for each student, and then mean attitude score toward each question was obtained. As Maximum point of Likert scale allotted to each question was 5(Strongly Agree), so overall attitude score of 8 questions is 5*8 = 40.

2.4 Statistical analysis

(IBM SPSS Version 23). The result was expressed in terms of frequency, percentage, mean, and SD.

**Ethical Consideration*: Ethical permission to conduct the study was sought from the IEC of Tripura Medical College & Dr. BRAM Teaching Hospital.

3. Results

Eighty-seven students took part in the study. Out of 87 students, 53 (61%) were females, while 34 (39%) were male participants (**Figure 1**).

We found that 71% of students had an attitude score > 35, while 29% of students had an attitude score ≤ 35 (**Figure 2**).

Ninety five percent of students agreed that CBME helped them learn better. More than 80% of students showed positive responses to all questions related to CBME (**Table 1**).

Mean attitude score of the students to every question ranged between 4.4 and 5, with all students (Mean 5 ± 0) agreeing with the easy learning concept of the CBME Curriculum (**Table 2**).

Out of a total (87*8) = 696 responses, 64.1% of students strongly agreed regarding the benefits of AETCOM, 33.5% agreed, while 2.2% of students showed neutral opinion and disagreed with 0.02% students (**Figure 3**).

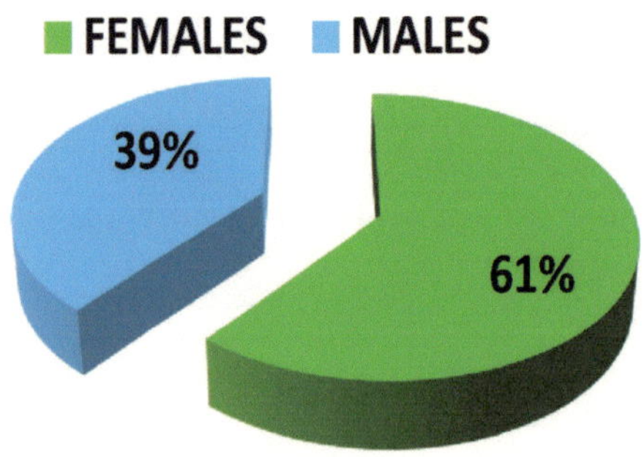

Figure 1.
Gender distribution of study participants.

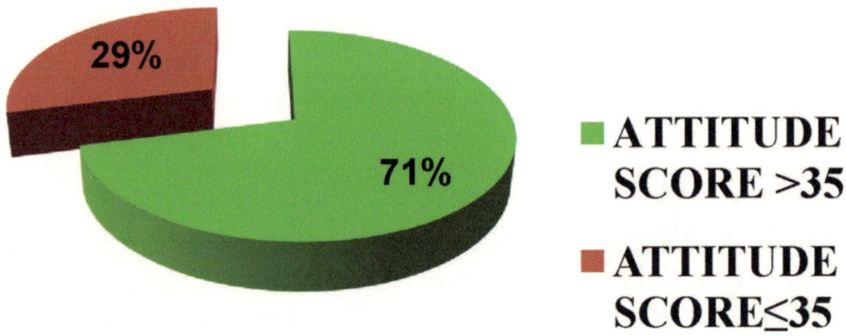

Figure 2.
Distribution of attitude score of the students.

Questions	No. of positive response (%)	No. of negative response (%)
Real-life situation	85(97.7%)	2(2.3%)
Help learning better	83(95.4%)	4(4.6%)
Relevance	85(97.7%)	2(2.3%)
Easy learning	87(100%)	0(0%)
Can improve participation	83(95.4%)	4(4.6%)
Helps gain competencies	86(98.8%)	1(1.2%)
Enjoyable	86(98.8%)	1(1.2%)
Preference for more AETCOM	84(96.5%)	3(3.5%)

Table 1.
Distribution of positive and negative responses to questions about CBME curriculum.

Question	Mean	SD	P value
Real-life situation	4.402298851	0.57989	0.00
HELPED learning better	4.528735632	0.625784725	
Relevance	4.666666667	0.520881781	
Easy learning	5	0	
Improve participation	4.597701149	0.579891131	
Helps gain competencies	4.551724138	0.522930488	
Enjoyable	4.517241379	0.525225731	
Preference for more AETCOM	4.643678	0.549355	

Table 2.
Mean score of all questions based on reflections from students.

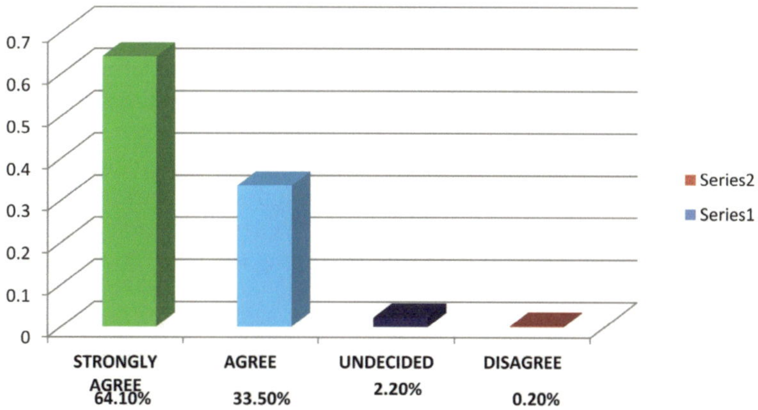

Figure 3.
Total distribution of responses of students.

4. Discussion

Total number of participants in our study was 87. As the study aims to find out the opinion of first professional MBBS students regarding the usefulness of AETCOM module 1.3, negative responses were also welcome. Out of a total attitude score of 40, all attitude scores of students ranged between 30 and 40; therefore, two groups were made, with 1 group having an attitude score ≤ 35 (having some neutral and negative responses) and another group of attitude score > 35 (having more positive responses).

We found that 71% of students had an attitude score > 35, while 29% of students had an attitude score ≤ 35. Our study findings were similar to a study conducted in Jhalawar Medical College where the vast majority of students (95%) had positive perceptions about the AETCOM-based CBME curriculum. This may be because the module helped them to understand the rights of patients, to communicate effectively with patients, and to develop the professional qualities and roles of a physician [6].

In our study, 95% of students gave an opinion post-class that AETCOM 1.3 helped them learn better. In a study of 2018,it was observed that observed that CBME is a useful method for a basic science like Physiology, and when combined with the traditional teaching method, can be retained and later practically applied [7]. Majority (>90% of participants) in our study felt that AETCOM module 1.3 would definitely help them improve their behavior toward patients. This was similar to a study done in Delhi where they found that 73% of medical students agreed the same following exposure to AETCOM modules [8].

Komattil R et al. in their study stated that students rated the module as "highly relevant" to the medical profession [9]. This was consistent with our study, as around 97% of our study participants gave the same opinion. Pandya et al. [10] stated that real-life personal experiences after AETCOM narratives, made it easier for students to encounter in the wards or clinics.

Similar was observed in a study done by Dhaliwal et al., 2018 in Delhi [11]. Shilpa et al. found in their study that AETCOM sessions helped students understand the term empathy for a good doctor-patient relationship and its role in effective patient management. Majority of our study participants also opined that the AETCOM module helped them develop ethics, communication, and professionalism [12].

Study by Vijayasree et al. in 2019 [13] observed that their study participants found AETCOM module 1.3 to be extremely promising, which would definitely improve their communication skills with patients. More than 95% of students in our study also had a similar opinion.

Earlier studies regarding the implementation of AETCOM included the perceptions of the faculty members [14, 15]. Ours is among few that include [16] the perception of medical undergraduates regarding the usefulness of AETCOM 1.3 in the undergraduate medical curriculum for developing the base for strong clinical practice [17].

The bound environment of med schools leads to challenges in newer module introductions compared to traditional teaching methods [18]. Also, a "Good Student" based on the marking system might not be a "Good Doctor" [19, 20]. Thus, AETCOM targets all students to develop their moral behavior, and there lies the motivation and importance of learning AETCOM module 1.3, that is, Doctor-Patient Relationship [20].

Overall, it can be recommended that Teaching of AETCOM module 1.3 could serve as an effective medium to teach students about issues and ethical practices and to understand the professional qualities and roles of a physician that are not conventionally taught in the Physiology core curriculum.

5. Limitations of the study

Students were asked to give their genuine opinions through reflective notes without revealing their name and roll number; nevertheless, the chances of bias could not be ruled out. Also, as only 87 students met the inclusion criteria, a large sample size could not be obtained for such a study.

6. Future scope

Studies regarding formative and summative assessments can be carried out through questions from AETCOM modules, and their scores may be compared with exam scores of Physiology core lecture classes.

7. Conclusion

It can be concluded that formal training in AETCOM competencies has a positive effect on shaping the professional attitudes of medical students. Role plays and clinical exposure are perceived as effective ways of imparting ethics education. This positive effect can be enhanced with improved teaching-learning methods for successive batches of undergraduate medical trainees. Thus, teaching-learning of AETCOM module 1.3 is one of the most effective ways for students to develop communication skills, doctor-patient relationships and to understand the professional qualities and roles of a physician.

Author details

Abirlal Sen[1]*, Manidipa Barman[2] and Sarjubala Thingujam[3]

1 Department of Physiology, Tripura Medical College and Dr. BRAM Teaching Hospital, Agartala, Tripura, India

2 Department of Pediatrics, Tripura Medical College and Dr. BRAM Teaching Hospital, Agartala, Tripura, India

3 Department of Obstetrics and Gynaecology, NEIGRIHMS, Shillong, Meghalaya, India

*Address all correspondence to: drabirlalsen@gmail.com

References

[1] National Medical Commission. Information Desk – For Colleges – UG Curriculum. Available from: https://www.nmc.org.in/information-desk/for-colleges/ug-curriculum/. [Last accessed on 2025 April 30]

[2] Barde PB, Patel D, Kathrotia R, Sharma G, Chitturi V, Parmar N, et al. Teaching of AETCOM modules in Physiology using Peer assisted learning: Feasibility assessment study. Indian Journal of Physiology and Allied Sciences. 2022;**74**(1). DOI: 10.55184/ijpas.v74i1.36

[3] Amarantha DR, Noor T, Swanand SP. Effect of Education in AETCOM Competencies in Shaping the Professional Attitudes of Medical Students. South-East Asian Journal of Medical Education. 30 Dec 2022;**16**(2)

[4] National Medical Commission. Information Desk – For Colleges – UG Curriculum. Available from: https://www.nmc.org.in/wp-content/uploads/2020/01/AETCOM_book.pdf [Last accessed on 2025 April 30]

[5] Harpe SE. How to analyze Likert and other rating scale data. Currents in Pharmacy Teaching and Learning. 2015;**7**:836-850. DOI: 10.1016/j.cptl.2015.08.001

[6] Verma A, Shete S. Perceptions of 1st-year MBBS students and 1st-year medical faculties toward AETCOM-based medical curriculum. National Journal of Physiology, Pharmacy & Pharmacology. 1 Mar 2024;**14**(3)

[7] Shah C. Early clinical exposure-why and how? Journal of Education Technology in Health Sciences. 2018;**5**(1):2-7

[8] Gurtoo A, Ranjan P, Sud R, Kumari A. A study of acceptability & feasibility of integrating humanities based study modules in undergraduate curriculum. The Indian Journal of Medical Research. 2013;**137**(1):197

[9] Komattil R, Hande SH, Mohammed CA, Subramaniam B. Evaluation of a personal and professional development module in an undergraduate medical curriculum in India. Korean Journal of Medical Education. 2016;**28**(1):117

[10] Pandya R, Shukla R, Gor AP, Ganguly B. Personal experience narratives by students: A teaching-learning tool in bioethics. Indian Journal of Medical Ethics. 2016;**1**(3):144-147

[11] Dhaliwal U, Singh S, Singh N. Reflective student narratives: Honing professionalism and empathy. Indian Journal of Medical Ethics. 2018;**3**(1):9-15

[12] Shilpa M, Raghunandana R, Narayana K. Empathy in medical education: Does it need to be taught? Students feedback on AETCOM module of learning. National Journal of Physiology, Pharmacy and Pharmacology. 2021;**11**(4):401-405

[13] Vijayasree M. Perception of attitude, ethics and communication skills (AETCOM) module by first MBBS students as a learning tool in the foundation course. Journal of Evidence-Based Medicine and Healthcare. 2019;**6**(42):2750-2753

[14] Ghosh A, Bir A. Role of written examination in the assessment of attitude ethics and communication in medical students: Perceptions of medical

faculties. Journal of Education Health Promotion. 2021;**10**:23

[15] Soundariya K, Kalaiselvan G, Rajalakshmi M, Sindhuri R. Implementation and evaluation of competency-based medical education in phase I of undergraduate medical curriculum. Journal of Advances in Medical Education & Professionalism. 2022;**10**:228-234

[16] Jain T, Mohan Y, Maiya GR, Nesan GS, Boominathan C, Eashwar AV. Evaluating the effectiveness of 'AETCOM module' on the medical interns posted in peripheral health centres of a tertiary care medical college in Kanchipuram, Tamil Nadu. Journal of Family Medicine and Primary Care. 2022;**11**:2828-2833

[17] Sharma V, Aggarwal M, Kumari P, Parashar L, Bhati RK, Singh A, et al. Impact of AETCOM module about autonomy, empathy and equanimity on ensuing clinical practice: Perceptions of medical undergraduates. Indian Journal of Physiology and Pharmacology. 2024;**68**:344-349. DOI: 10.25259/IJPP_346_2023

[18] Rajashree R, Chandrashekar DM. Competency-based medical education in [14] India: A work in progress. Indian Journal of Physiology and Pharmacology. 2020;**64**(1):57-59

[19] Tikare S. Reflective writing: Experience of first professional medical students with [20] attitude ethics and communication module. South-East Asian Journal of Medical Education. 2021;**15**(1):41-49

[20] Corinne T, Neville C, Anna R. Perceived educational impact of the medical [22] student long case: A qualitative study. BMC Medical Education. 2020;**20**:257-258

Section 3

Advanced Topics in Medical Education

Chapter 5

Dismantling Bias in Medical Education: Redefining Training by Removing Race-Based Frameworks

Antoinette Leonard-Jean Charles

Abstract

This chapter explores the urgent need to dismantle race-based frameworks in medical education and clinical practice. It critiques the historical influence of the Flexner Report and other entrenched biases that have shaped medical curricula, resulting in training models that often perpetuate racial stereotypes and systemic disparities in patient care. By analyzing the limitations of race-based medicine and advocating for a shift toward evidence-based, bias-free frameworks, this chapter presents an approach to reorienting medical education toward health equity. It also outlines actionable steps for academic medicine leaders to implement curricula that prioritize cultural competency, structural competency, and individualized patient care over outdated racial assumptions. Ultimately, this chapter argues that by removing biased frameworks, medical education can produce physicians who advocate for all communities, are equipped to address the social determinants of health and deliver truly inclusive, patient-centered care. The persistence of race-based frameworks in medical education perpetuates systemic disparities and biased clinical practices. Especially when the age person is more than one race or ethnicity, moreover race has no biologically implication. This chapter critically examines the historical roots and ongoing impact of race-based medicine, mainly influenced by the Flexner Report of 1910, which led to the marginalization of minority-serving institutions and embedded racial biases into medical training. The chapter advocates for an evidence-based approach that prioritizes structural and cultural competency while eliminating race as a biological determinant in medical curricula. Strategies for curriculum reform and institutional change are presented to foster a more equitable and inclusive healthcare system.

Keywords: medical education reform, race-based medicine, bias in healthcare, cultural competency, health equity

1. Introduction

The legacy of race-based medicine, deeply embedded in the historical foundations of the standardization of medical education and practice, continues to perpetuate health disparities and systemic biases [1]. Rooted in the early twentieth century, particularly influenced by the Flexner Report of 1910 [2–5], medical training in the United States established a framework that often [6, 7] conflated biological determinism with racial categorization [2, 6, 8–10]. Leading to harmful assumptions about health and disease based on race rather than evidence-based science or individualized care [6, 9] While initially framed as scientific progress, this approach has reinforced inequities, impacting the diagnosis, treatment, and outcomes of historically marginalized communities.

Recent scholarship highlights the urgent need to critique these race-based frameworks and pivot toward a bias-free medical curriculum that aligns with modern scientific understanding. Racial categorizations, though historically convenient, have proven to be both scientifically inaccurate and socially harmful. Instead, a shift toward curricula that emphasize genetics, social determinants of health, and personalized medicine is necessary to address disparities effectively [5, 11]. This approach recognizes the complexity of health beyond racial binaries, advocating for systems that assess patients' needs based on individual and contextual factors rather than predetermined racial assumptions.

In addition to curriculum changes, the development of structural competency and cultural sensitivity is critical for equipping physicians with tools to address health inequities without relying on racial categorization. Structural competency emphasizes understanding the societal and systemic factors; such as poverty, access to care, and environmental conditions that influence health outcomes [12, 13]. Integrating this into medical education can enable future physicians to critically engage with the root causes of disparities rather than perpetuating racial stereotypes in practice.

However, systemic transformation requires institutional change beyond curriculum adjustments. Academic leaders play a pivotal role in facilitating this shift, through strategies such as faculty education, implementation of race-free assessment tools, and creation of anti-racist policies within medical schools [14, 15]. Such reforms are necessary to dismantle entrenched biases, promote equity, and prepare healthcare providers to deliver care that is truly patient-centered and just.

This chapter aims to critically analyze the historical underpinnings of race-based medicine, propose evidence-based curricular reforms, outline strategies for cultural and structural competency training, and explore institutional pathways toward bias-free medical education. By addressing these interconnected objectives, the discussion seeks to contribute to a growing body of scholarship advocating for a healthcare system rooted in fairness, accuracy, and inclusivity.

2. The legacy of the Flexner report

Abraham Flexner, an influential educator and reformer with strong affiliations to the Carnegie Foundation, the Rockefeller Foundation, and Johns Hopkins University, significantly influenced the trajectory of medical education in the United States [7]. Tasked by the Carnegie Foundation with support from the Rockefeller Foundation, Flexner sought to overhaul medical education based on rigorous scientific principles. His recommendations led to the closure of numerous medical schools, particularly those serving Black and minority communities, under the pretext of standardization and modernization [7]. Flexner's work, while intended to professionalize the field, disproportionately impacted marginalized communities and perpetuated systemic inequities that continue to affect healthcare access and outcomes today [3, 6, 9].

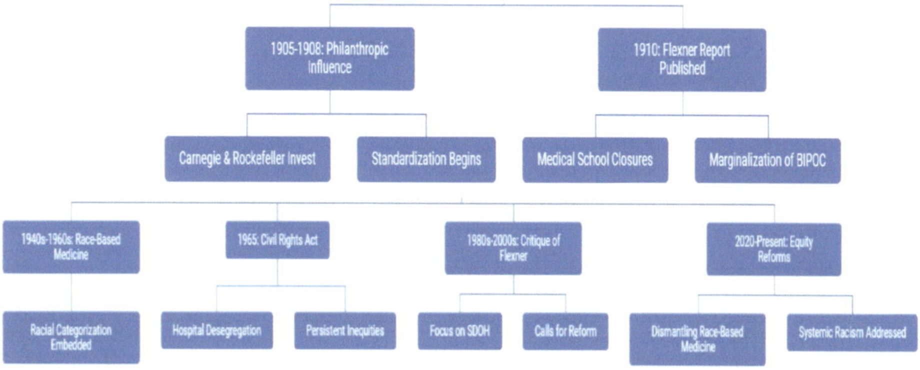

Figure 1.
Historical timeline of Race in medicine.

The Flexner Report of 1910 institutionalized an exclusionary framework that prioritized elite, predominantly white institutions, reinforcing barriers for BIPOC communities in medical education and clinical practice. The closure of historically Black medical schools significantly reduced opportunities for Black physicians, exacerbating racial health disparities that persist into the present era. The legacy of the report remains deeply ingrained in medical curricula, influencing policies that shape healthcare education and delivery. Addressing the enduring impact of Flexner's reforms requires deliberate efforts to dismantle systemic biases and foster a more inclusive and representative healthcare workforce (**Figure 1**).

3. Methodology

The chapter is a systematic literature historical review. An extension of the recent work of my dissertation, *Unmasking The Nexus of the Nexus of Race, Education, and Health: An Intersectional Analysis of Epistemology of Race in Medicine, Medical Curricula, and Health Disparities*. Much of the methodology used in the study was conducted to critically analyze the role of race-based frameworks in medical education and propose reforms centered on structural and cultural competency. Data were collected from reputable electronic databases, including PubMed, Google Scholar, and Scopus, to ensure comprehensive coverage of peer-reviewed publications. The search strategy employed a combination of keywords such as "race-based medicine," "structural competency," "health equity," and "medical curriculum reform" to capture relevant studies and discussions. A thematic analysis approach was employed to highlight key challenges and opportunities for reform, with an emphasis on evidence-based strategies to foster equitable healthcare training.

3.1 Inclusion criteria

The review included studies that met the following criteria: Peer-reviewed articles published between 2000 and the present. Articles examining the historical and contemporary impact of race-based medical frameworks. Studies focusing on educational interventions aimed at addressing racial biases in medical training. Publications in English to ensure accessibility and relevance to the target audience.

3.2 Exclusion criteria

Studies were excluded based on the following criteria: Non-peer-reviewed sources, including opinion pieces and editorial articles. Articles lacking empirical data or clear methodological frameworks. Studies published in languages other than English.

4. Historical context of race-based medicine

The persistence of race-based medicine within healthcare and medical education is deeply rooted in historical frameworks that continue to influence modern practice. Among these legacies, the Flexner Report of 1910 played a pivotal role in standardizing medical education while simultaneously exacerbating systemic inequities. This report, though instrumental in advancing scientific rigor, marginalized medical institutions that served Black, Indigenous, and People of Color (BIPOC) communities and further entrenched racial biases within clinical training and practice [16, 17]. By closing the majority of historically Black medical schools, the Flexner Report significantly reduced the number of Black physicians, creating long-term gaps in healthcare access for Black communities, a disparity that persists today. This exclusion has had generational impacts, not only in terms of access to care but also in the underrepresentation of BIPOC individuals in medical leadership and policymaking, which has perpetuated the narrow, exclusionary approach to healthcare delivery [2]. These biases not only impacted the enrollment and retention of diverse populations in medical education but also solidified a narrow, exclusionary approach to healthcare delivery—one that perpetuates disparities for BIPOC and LGBTQIA communities. To fully address the present-day impacts, it is essential to critically examine the historical underpinnings of race-based practices in clinical training, the flawed concept of race as a biological marker, and the far-reaching consequences of these biases on health outcomes for marginalized populations.

The remnants of race-based medicine continue to exist in diagnostic and treatment practices. A prominent example is the use of race-corrected algorithms in clinical tools such as the eGFR (estimated glomerular filtration rate), which adjusts kidney function estimates for Black patients under the false assumption that Black individuals have higher muscle mass and therefore higher creatinine levels. This adjustment often delays referrals for nephrology care, kidney transplants, and other critical treatments for Black patients, contributing to poorer health outcomes and increased mortality [1]. Similarly, race-based spirometry, used to assess lung function, incorporates adjustments for Black and Asian patients, rooted in outdated beliefs about inherent differences in lung capacity. This practice can mask the severity of respiratory conditions in these populations, delaying interventions and perpetuating disparities in respiratory health [18].

Another deeply concerning example of race-based bias is the enduring misconception that Black patients have a higher pain tolerance compared to white patients. This bias has been documented in numerous studies, where Black patients are less likely to receive appropriate pain management, such as opioid prescriptions, compared to white patients presenting with the same symptoms [10, 19]. Such beliefs stem from pseudoscientific ideas from the nineteenth century and continue to influence provider decision-making, resulting in undertreatment and poorer outcomes for Black patients experiencing pain. For instance, in emergency departments, Black and

Hispanic patients are consistently undertreated for acute pain compared to white patients, a disparity that further erodes trust in the healthcare system [2].

In addition, the lack of diversity in clinical research exacerbates these issues, as BIPOC and LGBTQIA populations are underrepresented in clinical trials, leading to treatment guidelines that do not account for their specific needs. For example, oncology treatments and cardiovascular therapies have historically been tested on predominantly white male populations, limiting their efficacy and safety for diverse groups [20]. This systemic bias within research contributes to inequities in treatment outcomes and further marginalizes populations that already experience barriers to care.

These practices illustrate how race-based medicine, while often framed as evidence-based, continues to perpetuate harm by embedding systemic bias into diagnostic tools, clinical decision-making, and medical research. As a result, BIPOC and LGBTQIA patients frequently experience delayed diagnoses, inadequate treatments, and higher rates of preventable complications and mortality compared to their white counterparts. Addressing these inequities requires a fundamental rethinking of medical education and clinical practice, with an emphasis on structural competency and anti-racist reforms to eliminate the misuse of race in healthcare. Systemic racism remains a driving force behind these disparities, as it shapes how race has historically been misinterpreted as a biological marker rather than a social construct. This flawed conceptualization has led to widespread biases in clinical decision-making, influencing diagnostic protocols, treatment guidelines, and patient-provider interactions in ways that perpetuate inequitable health outcomes.

4.1 Examination of race-based practices in clinical training and diagnosis through critical race theory (CRT)

Critical Race Theory (CRT) provides a vital lens for understanding the systemic inequities embedded in medical education and clinical training. By highlighting the intersections of race, power, and healthcare systems, CRT exposes how race-based practices became institutionalized. The Flexner Report serves as a foundational example of such practices, as its recommendations led to the closure of many historically Black medical schools, reducing the number of Black physicians and undermining healthcare access for marginalized populations [16, 21]. Flexner's emphasis on "scientific" medicine disproportionately favored predominantly white institutions while dismissing the culturally informed and community-based approaches of minority-serving schools [20, 21].

These systemic decisions influenced clinical training curricula, where racial stereotypes and biases were often perpetuated under the guise of medical science. For instance, race-based diagnostic tools and teaching practices continue to reinforce inaccurate assumptions, such as the use of race correction in clinical algorithms for kidney function and lung capacity. Such frameworks disregard the social and environmental determinants of health and instead rely on race as a flawed biological marker, ultimately marginalizing BIPOC patients. Moreover, these practices limit the perspectives included in clinical training, thereby fostering internal biases among healthcare providers who may lack awareness of the systemic factors influencing patient outcomes [18, 20].

4.2 Race as a biological marker and systemic biases

The historical framing of race as a biological determinant of health is a direct consequence of colonial and post-Flexner medical practices [6, 7, 9]. This biological determinism assumes inherent racial differences in physiology and pathology, leading to systemic biases that persist today. The work of scholars such as Roberts [22] and Bonham et al. [23] underscores how race is a social construct that has been misinterpreted as a biological reality, influencing medical research, clinical guidelines, and healthcare delivery.

For example, the continued use of race-based medicine, such as adjustments for Black patients in estimated glomerular filtration rate (eGFR) calculations, reflects outdated notions of racial difference and contributes to disparities in diagnosis and treatment [1, 24]. Such practices can delay critical interventions, leading to worse outcomes for BIPOC populations. Similarly, reliance on racial categorization in clinical guidelines ignores the impact of social determinants of health, such as socioeconomic status, environmental exposures, and access to care, which are far more predictive of health outcomes than race itself [12, 20].

The systemic embedding of race as a biological marker has further implications for medical education. It discourages the inclusion of diverse perspectives and reinforces a culture of exclusion that limits innovation in research and clinical practice. For BIPOC and LGBTQIA populations, this creates barriers to enrollment, acceptance, and retention in medical programs, as these systems often fail to recognize or address the experiences and needs of marginalized students [25]. Without diversity in medical education, the field lacks the lived experiences necessary to challenge these biases and create more equitable healthcare systems.

4.3 Impact of systemic biases on health outcomes for BIPOC populations

The historical perpetuation of race-based medicine has resulted in measurable and persistent disparities in health outcomes for BIPOC and LGBTQIA populations. The reduction in diverse physician representation, stemming from the Flexner Report's impact on Black medical schools, has limited access to culturally competent care for marginalized communities [16, 17]. Research consistently shows that patients treated by physicians who share their racial or cultural background experience better communication, trust, and health outcomes [10, 26]. This alignment fosters greater cultural understanding, enabling providers to recognize and address nuanced patient concerns that might otherwise be overlooked [26]. In contrast, the lack of diversity among providers often leads to implicit biases, misinterpretation of symptoms, and clinical differential observer bias, where diagnostic decisions are influenced by racialized assumptions rather than clinical evidence [27]. These biases can result in treatment plans that inadequately address the specific needs of patients from BIPOC and LGBTQIA communities, further eroding trust and perpetuating health disparities. Expanding the diversity of the healthcare workforce is thus critical for building equitable and inclusive patient-provider relationships. Systemic racism underpins these disparities, shaping how race has historically been misused as a biological marker in clinical frameworks and perpetuating inequitable practices in healthcare delivery [28].

Systemic biases in medical education and practice have exacerbated disparities in mortality, chronic disease prevalence, and access to preventive care. For example, racialized assumptions about pain tolerance among Black patients have led to the undertreatment of pain, contributing to worse long-term health outcomes [19]. LGBTQIA population faces unique but similar barriers, including discrimination and inadequate provider training, leading to poorer mental and physical health outcomes. Many providers lack the competence necessary to understand the specific health needs of LGBTQIA individuals, resulting in miscommunication, discomfort, and avoidance of care by patients. Additionally, stigmatization and structural exclusion within healthcare systems often mean that LGBTQIA individuals face delayed diagnoses, limited access to affirming care, and suboptimal treatment outcomes compared to their heterosexual and cisgender counterparts [22, 25].

Addressing these disparities requires systemic reforms in medical education that prioritize inclusive curricula and equip healthcare providers with the tools to deliver equitable, culturally competent care. This leads directly to the need for Strategies to Improve Curriculum and Structural Competency, where targeted interventions can dismantle these long-standing inequities [12, 29].

4.4 Strategies to improve curriculum and structural competency

With these inequities, academic leaders must take decisive steps to revise clinical training as well as medical education especially since the US majority of medical institutions have combined clinical and medical education. Introducing anti-racist curricula and emphasizing structural competency, enables healthcare professionals to critically engage with systemic inequities rather than perpetuating racialized diagnoses [25]. A central approach involves introducing anti-racist curricula that challenge racialized frameworks in clinical training. These curricula should include critical examinations of the historical and sociopolitical factors that have shaped healthcare disparities, such as the enduring impact of the Flexner Report on marginalized communities [2, 16]. Integrating concepts from Critical Race Theory (CRT) into medical education, institutions can provide learners with tools to critically analyze systemic inequities in healthcare and reject flawed practices such as race-based diagnostic algorithms [18, 27]. Furthermore, curricula must explicitly address the social determinants of health, highlighting how poverty, housing instability, and access to care are more influential predictors of health outcomes than race itself [12].

Structural competency must also be emphasized as a core component of medical education to equip future healthcare providers with the skills to identify and address systemic inequities. Metzl and Hansen [25] argue that structural competency goes beyond cultural competency by focusing on the larger structural forces—such as policies, institutions, and systems that shape individual and community health. To integrate this approach, medical curricula should include case-based learning and simulations that encourage students to examine the broader societal factors contributing to health disparities. For instance, structural competency training might involve analyzing real-world case studies that connect housing policies to asthma rates in urban BIPOC communities or exploring how food deserts contribute to diabetes prevalence among marginalized populations [10, 30]. Such educational approaches not only build awareness but also promote actionable solutions that address inequities at both systemic and clinical levels.

Another key strategy for improving curricula involves the inclusion of historically marginalized voices and experiences in medical education. Diverse representation among faculty, guest speakers, and standardized patients can provide students with critical insights into the lived experiences of BIPOC and LGBTQIA populations [2, 31]. Institutions should actively recruit and retain faculty members from underrepresented backgrounds and create mentorship programs to support students and educators alike. Incorporating community-led teaching initiatives, such as partnerships with organizations that serve marginalized populations, can further enrich students' understanding of structural inequities and improve their ability to deliver equitable care. Such initiatives not only combat internal biases but also promote trust between healthcare providers and the communities they serve [32].

Furthermore, revising assessment tools and clinical guidelines to eliminate race-based adjustments is crucial for ensuring equity in medical training and practice. Faculty education programs must focus on deconstructing implicit biases and re-examining diagnostic protocols that rely on race as a proxy for biological differences [1]. For example, the use of race-neutral equations in renal function assessment has been proposed to replace eGFR algorithms that inaccurately adjust for Black patients, which delay referrals for critical treatments [33]. Updated guidelines must prioritize individualized care rooted in genetics, lifestyle factors, and social determinants of health rather than outdated and harmful racial categories. Faculty development workshops, ongoing implicit bias training, and updated curricular materials can ensure that educators are equipped to teach these revised practices effectively [14, 34].

These strategies collectively aim to dismantle the systemic roots of race-based medicine while promoting structural competency and anti-racist medical education. By integrating these reforms, academic leaders can prepare future healthcare providers to engage critically with inequities and deliver patient-centered, equitable care. While revising medical curricula and fostering structural competency represent crucial steps in eliminating systemic biases, addressing the flawed conceptualization of race as a biological marker remains central to this effort. Historically, race has been misused in clinical practice and research as a biological determinant of health, leading to widespread systemic biases. The next section will explore how this misconception continues to impact diagnostic practices, perpetuate inequities, and produce harmful health outcomes for BIPOC and LGBTQIA populations.

5. Critique of current race-based frameworks

Race-based frameworks remain deeply entrenched in modern medical practice, influencing diagnoses, treatment protocols, and healthcare delivery. One prominent example includes the use of race as a variable in clinical decision-making tools, such as the race-based adjustments in estimated glomerular filtration rate (eGFR) for kidney function and spirometry for lung health. These adjustments are rooted in historical pseudoscientific assumptions that falsely attribute biological differences to race, rather than acknowledging social, environmental, and genetic factors that shape health outcomes [1]. For instance, race-based spirometry adjusts predicted lung function downward for Black and Asian patients, which can mask disease severity and delay treatment for respiratory conditions [18]. Similarly, race-based eGFR values often delay access to life-saving interventions such as dialysis or kidney transplantation for Black patients, perpetuating disparities in renal care outcomes. These frameworks exemplify how racial categorization in clinical practice prioritizes flawed biological assumptions over patient-centered care, contributing to worse outcomes for BIPOC populations [26, 28, 35].

The harm caused by race-based assumptions in healthcare is particularly evident in maternal-fetal health outcomes. The decline or elimination of midwifery in the early twentieth century, largely driven by the rise of obstetrics and gynecology (OB/GYN) as a dominant medical specialty, had profound implications for BIPOC communities. Historically, midwives—many of whom were Black or Indigenous—provided culturally competent and community-based care to marginalized populations [16]. However, the Flexner Report's push for standardized medical education systematically excluded midwives and dismantled traditional care models, particularly those outside institutional settings [17]. This shift disproportionately impacted maternal health outcomes for Black and Indigenous women, who faced higher mortality rates due to structural inequities, lack of access to care, and implicit biases within the OB/GYN medical framework [2]. These disparities persist today, as Black women in the United States are nearly three times more likely to die from pregnancy-related complications compared to white women, a result of both systemic racism and the continued absence of culturally sensitive care models.

Another example the loss of private and community-based medical practices over the past two generations has exacerbated gaps in healthcare access for BIPOC and LGBTQIA populations. Historically, private practitioners, particularly in underserved communities, played a vital role in delivering culturally responsive care. However, the consolidation of healthcare systems into large hospital networks and the rising costs of medical education have reduced opportunities for physicians to practice independently, disproportionately affecting BIPOC and LGBTQIA providers and the communities they serve [2, 16, 36, 37]. This decline has resulted in fragmented care delivery, diminished patient-provider trust, and poorer health outcomes, particularly for marginalized populations who often feel overlooked or stigmatized within institutional healthcare settings.

Race-based frameworks reinforce these biases in clinical decision-making by normalizing racial categorization as a proxy for understanding health disparities. This practice overlooks the influence of social determinants, such as socioeconomic status, housing, education, and systemic racism, which are far more significant predictors of health outcomes than race itself [12, 20]. Physicians trained under race-based models may unconsciously perpetuate inequities, as these frameworks fail to equip them with the tools to critically examine the structural and cultural factors that shape patient health. As a result, providers may develop treatment plans based on flawed assumptions rather than addressing the complex social realities of their patients, leading to suboptimal care and persistent disparities.

5.1 Integrating structural competency and cultural sensitivity

Medical education must prioritize structural competency and cultural sensitivity as core components of physician training. Structural competency moves beyond cultural competency by encouraging healthcare providers to analyze and address the systemic factors—such as policies, institutional structures, and socioeconomic conditions—that shape health outcomes [11, 22, 25, 29]. For example, physicians can be trained to identify how housing discrimination, food insecurity, and environmental exposures contribute to chronic illnesses in underserved populations. Integrating structural competency into clinical training requires case-based learning, simulations, and community partnerships that connect theoretical knowledge to real-world practice [10, 29, 38].

Equally important is fostering cultural sensitivity to ensure that physicians develop the interpersonal skills needed to engage meaningfully with patients from diverse backgrounds. Training programs should incorporate the lived experiences of BIPOC and LGBTQIA individuals through workshops, patient narratives, and collaboration with community organizations. This approach can reduce implicit bias, improve patient-provider communication, and promote trust, ultimately leading to better health outcomes [13, 39, 40]. By shifting from race-based frameworks to structural and culturally sensitive approaches, medical education can better prepare healthcare providers to address health disparities without relying on racial categorization. The integration of structural competency and cultural sensitivity represents a critical step toward dismantling race-based medicine. However, achieving meaningful change requires a systematic reform of medical curricula to ensure that future physicians are equipped with the knowledge and skills needed to deliver equitable, bias-free care. The following section will outline proposed curriculum reforms that center on social determinants of health, patient-centered care, and evidence-based frameworks.

6. Proposed curriculum reform

Shifting toward a bias-free medical education demands a comprehensive overhaul of curricula to replace race-based practices with evidence-based frameworks that emphasize genetics, environmental influences, and social determinants of health [41]. Such reform must also incorporate structural and cultural competency training to prepare future physicians to provide equitable and patient-centered care. This section outlines the critical components of a reimagined medical curriculum, focusing on transitioning to evidence-based frameworks, integrating cultural competency, and embedding structural competency into physician training [28].

6.1 Transition to evidence-based frameworks

Current medical curricula often group individuals by race when teaching illness and pathology, perpetuating misconceptions about biological determinism [30]. To counter this, a reformed curriculum must emphasize evidence-based frameworks that focus on genetics, regional influences, and environmental factors, which are scientifically valid predictors of health outcomes. For example, conditions such as *G6PD deficiency, thalassemia, and sickle cell anemia* originated as evolutionary adaptations in specific regions to protect populations from malaria. These conditions are not racial but are tied to genetic traits prevalent in individuals from malaria-endemic areas, such as parts of Africa, Southeast Asia, and the Mediterranean [19, 29, 37].

Epigenetic research highlights how environmental factors, such as diet, stress, and pollution, influence gene expression over time, affecting the risk of chronic diseases. For instance, disparities in bone density and muscle mass among BIPOC populations are linked to environmental exposure, such as varying levels of sunlight influencing vitamin D metabolism [3, 9, 16, 20]. Additionally, health differences based on sex and gender must be integrated into this framework, as men and women often present differently for conditions such as heart disease. Women, for example, are more likely to experience subtle symptoms such as nausea or fatigue in cardiac events, while men may exhibit classic chest pain. Training future physicians to recognize these nuances will ensure more accurate diagnoses and treatments for all patients, moving beyond reductive racial categorizations [13, 27, 40].

Instead of grouping populations by race, curricula should use genetic, regional, or ethnic classifications to better understand disease prevalence and presentation. For example, blood type distributions vary globally and have implications for transfusion medicine and disease susceptibility. These patterns are rooted in genetic and regional variation, not race, and provide a scientifically sound basis for medical education. While generalized grouping may still be problematic in the context of evolving understandings of epigenetics, these frameworks are a significant improvement over outdated race-based models.

6.2 Integrating competency

Competency must be woven into every stage of medical education to equip physicians with the tools to provide individualized care for diverse populations. This involves teaching students to understand and respect the cultural, social, and historical contexts that shape patient experiences and health outcomes. A culturally competent curriculum includes training on communication strategies, understanding implicit biases, and recognizing how societal factors such as discrimination and marginalization impact health [37].

Practical tools for embedding cultural competency into curricula include case studies, role-playing exercises, and standardized patient interactions that simulate encounters with individuals from various backgrounds. Faculty development programs are essential to ensure instructors are equipped to teach cultural sensitivity effectively. Workshops, webinars, and curated resource guides can provide faculty with the knowledge and confidence to facilitate meaningful discussions on cultural awareness and its impact on clinical care [4, 5, 9]. Incorporating these methods helps foster an environment where future physicians are prepared to engage with diverse patients empathetically and equitably.

Additionally, involving community voices in curriculum design can help medical schools address gaps in cultural competency. Engaging leaders from BIPOC and LGBTQIA communities, as well as patient advocates, ensures that medical training reflects the lived experiences and needs of these populations. This participatory approach promotes a deeper understanding of health inequities and empowers students to serve as agents of change within the healthcare system [14, 23].

6.3 Structural competency training

Structural competency expands the focus from individual cultural differences to the broader systemic forces that shape health outcomes, such as socioeconomic policies, institutional inequities, and environmental conditions [3, 6, 9, 34]. Training in structural competency prepares future physicians to critically examine how societal structures influence patient health and equip them to advocate for systemic change. For example, coursework could include analyses of how redlining policies have contributed to higher rates of asthma and hypertension in urban BIPOC communities, or how food deserts increase the prevalence of diabetes in underserved populations [14, 19, 31].

Experiential learning is a key component of structural competency training. Students can participate in community health initiatives, shadow healthcare providers in underserved areas, or engage in advocacy projects addressing public health disparities. Case studies that incorporate social determinants of health, such as housing insecurity or occupational hazards, encourage students to move beyond symptom-focused care and consider the systemic barriers their patients face [42]. These experiences not only deepen understanding but also foster a commitment to addressing inequities within the healthcare system.

Another effective strategy involves integrating structural competency into interprofessional education, where medical students collaborate with peers from social work, public health, and law to tackle complex health challenges. This multidisciplinary approach mirrors real-world healthcare delivery and underscores the interconnectedness of structural factors across sectors [13, 30]. By transitioning to evidence-based frameworks, integrating cultural competency, and embedding structural competency into curricula, medical education can begin to dismantle the harmful legacies of race-based medicine. However, achieving these reforms requires ongoing evaluation, adaptability, and collaboration among educators, students, and community stakeholders. In the next section, we explore how implementing these changes can redefine the future of medical education and ultimately contribute to more equitable health outcomes for all.

7. Implementation strategies for academic leaders

Achieving a meaningful transition from race-based frameworks to bias-free, evidence-based medical education requires deliberate, strategic efforts from academic leaders. Medical institutions must take practical steps to reform curricula, train faculty, and assess the outcomes of these changes [13, 25, 39]. This process begins with an acknowledgment of the historical and systemic roots of racial bias in medical education and the ways these biases continue to harm marginalized populations, including BIPOC and LGBTQIA communities. Institutional leaders must engage stakeholders at all levels—administrators, educators, students, and community representatives;to ensure reforms are comprehensive, sustainable, and reflective of the diverse populations they aim to serve. Furthermore, implementing these changes requires a commitment to continuous evaluation and adaptation, as equity in healthcare is a dynamic goal that evolves alongside advancements in medicine, genetics, and understanding of social determinants of health. By prioritizing anti-racist, evidence-based frameworks, medical institutions can foster an environment that prepares future physicians to deliver inclusive, patient-centered care. The following section outlines practical strategies for faculty training, curricular integration, and measuring the long-term impact of these reforms on medical education and patient outcomes.

7.1 Practical steps for medical institutions to adopt curriculum changes

Medical institutions must begin with a systematic audit of existing curricula to identify areas where race-based frameworks are embedded in teaching materials, clinical guidelines, and assessment practices. A curriculum task force comprising educators, students, clinicians, and community representatives can facilitate this process, ensuring that reforms are comprehensive and inclusive of diverse perspectives [27, 43]. For example, institutions should replace race-based clinical algorithms—such as race corrections in spirometry and eGFR—with race-neutral, evidence-based models grounded in genetics, social determinants, and regional factors [24, 32].

Curriculum redesign should also prioritize courses that teach physicians to critically examine systemic inequities, genetics, and environmental influences on health. This includes integrating modules on structural competency, social determinants of health, and cultural sensitivity into core medical training [25, 31]. Additionally, courses that emphasize epigenetics and evolutionary biology—for instance, understanding how G6PD deficiency, sickle cell disease, or thalassemia arose as genetic adaptations to protect regional populations from malaria—can provide a scientific foundation for understanding population-level health differences without relying on racial categorization [42, 44].

A key step in Integration includes securing institutional support from leadership downward, and horizontally into clinical practices. An essential for allocation of policy enforcement and profession development (retraining) and evaluation [25, 32, 35]. By aligning these reforms with broader institutional goals of equity and inclusion, academic leaders can foster a culture that prioritizes anti-bias education and evidence-based care.

7.2 Faculty training in anti-bias education and continuous assessment

Faculty members play a central role in implementing curriculum reforms and shaping the perspectives of future physicians. Therefore, it is essential to provide faculty with robust training in anti-bias education, cultural humility, and structural competency. Workshops, seminars, and ongoing professional development programs can equip faculty with the tools to recognize their own implicit biases and teach students to critically examine systemic inequities [7, 34].

One effective strategy involves integrating faculty development programs that focus on evidence-based teaching methods and anti-racist pedagogy. These programs should include case-based learning exercises, community engagement initiatives, and simulations that expose faculty to the lived experiences of marginalized populations [28, 41]. Faculty should also be trained to address topics such as regional genetics, gender differences in disease presentation, and the role of social determinants of health in shaping patient outcomes. For example, understanding the unique ways heart disease presents in women compared to men can challenge gendered biases in clinical decision-making [35].

Continuous assessment of faculty training is equally important. Regular evaluations, feedback loops, and peer reviews can help ensure that anti-bias education remains effective and aligned with evolving medical evidence and societal needs. Faculty must be supported with tools and resources, such as standardized teaching materials and evidence-based guidelines, to facilitate consistent and impactful instruction.

7.3 Strategies for measuring the impact of reforms on student outcomes and patient care

To assess the effectiveness of curriculum reforms, medical institutions must implement robust evaluation frameworks that measure both student learning outcomes and the long-term impact on patient care [29]. These frameworks should include a combination of quantitative and qualitative metrics to track progress over time.

At the student level, evaluations can focus on knowledge acquisition, clinical decision-making, and cultural humility. Tools such as standardized assessments, objective structured clinical examinations (OSCEs), and reflective portfolios can measure how well students are integrating evidence-based frameworks, structural competency, and cultural sensitivity into their practice [29, 30]. For example, case scenarios requiring students to address social determinants of health or consider genetic and regional factors in treatment decisions can assess their ability to move beyond racialized thinking.

To evaluate patient outcomes, institutions can collaborate with healthcare systems to track metrics such as improved care delivery, reduced diagnostic delays, and better patient satisfaction among BIPOC and LGBTQIA populations. Collecting data on patient-provider trust and health disparities in clinical outcomes can provide valuable insights into the real-world impact of these reforms [10, 11, 29].

Longitudinal studies and alumni surveys can also be used to assess how medical graduates apply anti-bias training and structural competency in their professional practice. These data can inform ongoing curriculum adjustments and demonstrate the value of evidence-based, bias-free education to institutional stakeholders and policymakers.

8. Aligning policy and practice

The implementation of these strategies has significant implications for both policy and clinical practice. By providing a concrete roadmap for eliminating race-based frameworks, academic leaders can transform medical education into a model of equity, accuracy, and inclusivity. Aligning these changes with broader institutional policies ensures that reforms are sustainable and actionable, influencing not only how future physicians are trained but also how they deliver care.

In the next section, we will explore the implications of these curriculum reforms for both healthcare systems and patient care outcomes, highlighting the practical applications of a bias-free, evidence-based approach to medical education.

9. Implementation strategies for academic leaders

The transition to bias-free medical education necessitates well-structured strategies that academic leaders can employ to effectively reform curricula, train faculty, and measure the outcomes of these changes. This effort aligns with the broader goal of dismantling race-based frameworks in healthcare and ensuring that future physicians are equipped with the tools to provide equitable and inclusive care. Below, we outline practical steps for medical institutions to implement these reforms, including faculty training in anti-bias education and strategies for evaluating the impact of these changes on both students and patient care.

9.1 Practical steps for medical institutions to adopt curriculum changes

Institutions must begin by conducting a comprehensive review of existing curricula to identify and eliminate areas where race-based frameworks persist. A curriculum review committee, composed of faculty, students, and community advocates, can analyze teaching materials, clinical case studies, and assessment tools to ensure they align with evidence-based, anti-racist principles [18, 39, 45]. This review should prioritize the removal of race-based clinical tools, such as race corrections in eGFR calculations, and their replacement with race-neutral models that emphasize social determinants of health and individual patient factors [28, 40].

Additionally, institutions can embed courses that focus on structural competency, cultural sensitivity, and epigenetics to address the root causes of health disparities. Case-based learning and small-group discussions on topics such as gender-specific symptoms of heart disease, genetic adaptations like G6PD deficiency, and the impact of environmental exposures on health should be included to provide students with a nuanced understanding of patient care [1, 25, 26]. Institutions should also create partnerships with local communities to incorporate real-world examples of systemic inequities and health disparities into classroom instruction [37].

Finally, securing institutional buy-in from leadership is critical to these reforms. Academic leaders must advocate for these changes at departmental and administrative levels, ensuring resources such as funding, faculty training, and updated teaching materials are available to support the transition [33].

9.2 Faculty training in anti-bias education and the importance of continuous assessment

Faculty are the cornerstone of effective curriculum reform, and their training in anti-bias education is essential for creating a bias-free learning environment. Comprehensive faculty development programs must focus on fostering self-awareness, addressing implicit biases, and teaching culturally sensitive approaches to healthcare. For example, workshops and training sessions can include simulations of clinical encounters with diverse patient populations, providing faculty with hands-on experience in addressing health disparities without relying on racial categorizations [22, 33].

To ensure consistency, institutions should establish peer mentoring programs where faculty can share best practices and receive constructive feedback on their teaching methods. This can be complemented by providing faculty with evidence-based resources and guidelines for structuring their lessons, such as updated clinical algorithms, case studies rooted in social determinants of health, and frameworks for understanding genetic and regional influences on disease prevalence [39, 40].

Continuous assessment of faculty training is equally important. Institutions can use tools such as faculty self-assessments, student feedback surveys, and periodic evaluations of teaching effectiveness to ensure faculty are meeting the goals of anti-bias education. These assessments should not only measure faculty understanding but also evaluate their ability to integrate equity-focused principles into their teaching practices [14, 41].

9.3 Strategies for measuring the impact of reforms on student outcomes and patient care

38To assess the success of these reforms, academic leaders must implement robust evaluation frameworks that capture both short-term and long-term outcomes. For students, tools such as Objective Structured Clinical Examinations (OSCEs) and reflective writing assignments can assess their ability to apply evidence-based, culturally sensitive approaches in clinical scenarios [14, 23]. Longitudinal tracking of graduates' performance in clinical practice, such as their ability to reduce diagnostic disparities and improve patient satisfaction among BIPOC and LGBTQIA populations, can provide valuable data on the effectiveness of anti-bias education [43].

For patient care, institutions should collaborate with healthcare systems to track metrics such as reductions in diagnostic delays, improved management of chronic conditions, and increased trust and satisfaction among marginalized patients. For example, evaluating changes in outcomes for conditions such as diabetes, hypertension, or maternal mortality among BIPOC populations can offer insights into how well these reforms translate into improved healthcare delivery [30, 33, 40].

In addition to quantitative metrics, qualitative feedback from students, faculty, and community stakeholders can help refine and adapt these reforms over time. Institutional leaders must also consider integrating these findings into policy decisions, advocating for systemic changes that extend beyond medical education to address broader inequities in healthcare systems [45]. By implementing these strategies, academic leaders can create an educational environment that prepares future physicians to address health disparities with equity and empathy. These reforms not only influence medical education but also hold the potential to transform healthcare delivery, policy, and practice at large, fostering a system that prioritizes patient-centered, bias-free care. In the next section, we will explore the broader implications of these changes for healthcare systems and the future of medical practice.

10. Challenges and considerations

Implementing bias-free, evidence-based reforms in medical education presents several challenges that academic leaders must navigate to achieve meaningful and sustainable change. Resistance to these changes can arise from entrenched practices, institutional inertia, and broader systemic barriers. Addressing these challenges requires strategic planning, engagement with stakeholders, and a commitment to fostering diversity and equity at all levels of the academic medical system.

10.1 Resistance to change within academic medicine

One of the most significant challenges is resistance from within academic medicine itself. Faculty and administrators accustomed to traditional race-based frameworks may be reluctant to adopt new methodologies that require significant shifts in teaching approaches and clinical practices. Additionally, there may be skepticism about the effectiveness of anti-bias training and structural competency modules, particularly among those who view these concepts as peripheral to medical education. Institutions can overcome this resistance by providing evidence-based data on the harms of race-based frameworks and the benefits of proposed changes. Faculty and administrative buy-in can also be facilitated through inclusive decision-making processes that involve educators, students, and community stakeholders from the start [1, 40].

Resistance may also come from students, particularly those who feel overwhelmed by the additional content focused on structural and cultural competencies. Engaging students through transparent communication about the relevance of these reforms to their future practice, along with incorporating active learning methods such as case-based scenarios, can mitigate pushback and encourage participation [11, 31, 45].

10.2 Addressing gaps in faculty expertise

Another challenge lies in gaps in current faculty expertise regarding cultural and structural competencies. Many educators were trained under traditional, race-based models and may lack the knowledge or confidence to teach these new frameworks effectively. Institutions must prioritize faculty development programs that include workshops, mentorship opportunities, and ongoing assessments to address these gaps [10] Partnering with external organizations and experts in structural competency and anti-bias education can further enhance faculty readiness. However, these programs require funding, time, and administrative support, which may be limited in some institutions.

10.3 Policy, legislative, and systemic barriers

Policy and legislative barriers can also hinder progress. In some regions, legislative efforts to limit discussions of systemic racism and equity in education may restrict the ability of institutions to implement anti-racist curricula fully [36]. Academic leaders must work closely with legal experts and advocacy groups to navigate these restrictions while finding innovative ways to integrate equity-focused training into broader curricular frameworks.

Systemic barriers also extend to admissions and hiring practices. Medical schools often struggle to recruit and retain diverse students and faculty due to long-standing inequities in education and professional pathways. The financial burden of medical education disproportionately affects students from BIPOC and LGBTQIA communities, limiting the diversity of applicants. Similarly, hiring practices often rely on traditional metrics, such as publication records, that may disadvantage candidates from underrepresented backgrounds [9, 12, 31] . Addressing these barriers requires targeted scholarship programs, mentorship initiatives, and active efforts to diversify hiring committees.

10.4 Limitations in available research

While significant progress has been made in understanding the harms of race-based medicine, gaps remain in the available research on the most effective ways to implement structural and cultural competency training [33, 36]. There is also limited longitudinal data on the impact of these reforms on patient outcomes and systemic inequities. Institutions must invest in continued study and evaluation, collaborating with healthcare systems and community partners to collect meaningful data [12].

10.5 Considerations for admissions, retention, and faculty hiring

Creating a pipeline for diversity at all levels of medical education and practice is critical for long-term change. Admissions processes must prioritize inclusivity, valuing diverse lived experiences and perspectives alongside traditional academic metrics. Retention efforts, such as mentorship programs and mental health resources, can support underrepresented students as they navigate the challenges of medical training [2, 6, 13, 26]. Similarly, hiring practices must move beyond tokenism, ensuring meaningful representation of BIPOC and LGBTQIA faculty in leadership roles and on decision-making committees [33, 36].

Addressing these challenges requires a coordinated, institution-wide commitment to equity and inclusivity. By fostering collaboration, investing in faculty development, and prioritizing diversity in admissions and hiring, medical schools can overcome resistance and systemic barriers. These efforts will not only enhance the effectiveness of curricular reforms but also ensure a more equitable future for medical education and healthcare delivery.

11. Conclusion

The removal of race-based frameworks from medical education is not only a moral imperative but a practical necessity for advancing healthcare equity and improving outcomes for all patients. Rooted in a flawed understanding of race as a biological determinant, these outdated frameworks have perpetuated systemic inequities, harmed marginalized populations, and limited the potential of medical education to deliver patient-centered care. Replacing them with evidence-based approaches focused on genetics, environmental factors, and social determinants of health provides a more accurate, equitable, and scientifically grounded foundation for teaching future physicians.

The proposed reforms—centered on transitioning to evidence-based frameworks, integrating cultural and structural competencies, and diversifying faculty and student bodies—have the potential to transform both the training of physicians and the care they provide. Future healthcare providers will be better equipped to recognize and address systemic inequities, reduce diagnostic and treatment disparities, and build trust with patients from diverse backgrounds. These changes can have a cascading effect, improving outcomes for historically underserved communities, fostering a culture of equity within healthcare systems, and driving broader societal change toward inclusivity and fairness in health outcomes.

For academic leaders and policymakers, the need for action is urgent. Institutions must take bold steps to revise curricula, train faculty in anti-bias and structural competencies, and measure the impact of these reforms on both students and patient care. Policymakers must support these efforts by ensuring that legislative and financial barriers do not impede the progress of equity-focused initiatives. Collaboration across educational institutions, healthcare systems, and community stakeholders will be essential to achieving these goals and sustaining them in the long term.

11.1 Future directions for research and writing

While this chapter provides a roadmap for eliminating race-based frameworks, several areas warrant further exploration and research:

1. *Longitudinal studies on reform outcomes:* Investigating the long-term impact of these curricular changes on patient outcomes, physician preparedness, and systemic health disparities.

2. *Expanding epigenetic research:* Exploring the interplay of genetics, environment, and social determinants to further refine evidence-based frameworks.

3. *Assessment of faculty development programs:* Evaluating the effectiveness of anti-bias and structural competency training for educators.

4. *Community-led health education models:* Researching the integration of community voices and lived experiences into medical curricula.

5. *Global perspectives on bias-free education:* Examining how these reforms can be adapted for medical education systems outside the United States, particularly in regions with unique healthcare challenges and disparities.

The journey to dismantle race-based frameworks in medical education is both challenging and necessary. By embracing evidence-based, equity-driven reforms, academic medicine has the opportunity to redefine its legacy, ensuring that future generations of physicians deliver care that is not only scientifically sound but also just and compassionate. Academic leaders and policymakers must take the lead in driving this critical transformation, ensuring that the healthcare system becomes a true model of equity and inclusion.

Author details

Antoinette Leonard-Jean Charles[1,2]

1 Long Island University, Brooklyn, NY, United States

2 Antioch University, Yellow Spring, Ohio, United States

*Address all correspondence to: antoinette.ljcharles@gmail.com

References

[1] Nieblas-Bedolla E, Christophers B, Nkinsi NT, Schumann PD, Stein E. Changing how race is portrayed in medical education: Recommendations from medical students. Academic Medicine. 2020;**95**(12):1802-1806. DOI: 10.1097/acm.0000000000003496

[2] Amutah C, Greenidge K, Mante A, Munyikwa M, Surya S, Higginbotham EJ, et al. Misrepresenting race — The role of medical schools in propagating physician bias. The New England Journal of Medicine. 2021;**384**(9):872-878. DOI: 10.1056/nejmms2025768

[3] Anderson N, Nguyen M, Marcotte K, Ramos M, Gruppen L, Boatright D. The long shadow: A historical perspective on racism in medical education. Academic Medicine. 2023;**98**(8S):S28-S36. DOI: 10.1097/acm.0000000000005253

[4] Asfaw Z, Barthélemy E. Anti-racist medical education in the transformation of global health. Tropical Doctor. 2022;**52**(2):245-245. DOI: 10.1177/00494755221077807

[5] Ayanian JZ, Williams R. Principles for eliminating racial and ethnic disparities in healthcare. In: Humana Press eBooks. 2007. pp. 377-389. DOI: 10.1007/978-1-59745-485-8_18

[6] Beck A. The Flexner report and the standardization of American medical education. JAMA. 2004;**291**(17):2139-2140. DOI: 10.1001/jama.291.17.2139

[7] Flexner A. Medical Education in the United States and Canada: A Report to the Carnegie Foundation for the Advancement of Teaching. 1910

[8] Ahmed A, Gittens B, Stewart S, Shalin S. Demographics and perceptions of diversity in the United States dermatopathology workforce and training environments. Journal of Cutaneous Pathology. 2022;**50**(4):330-337. DOI: 10.1111/cup.14347

[9] Bailey M. The Flexner report: Standardizing medical students through the region-, gender-, and race-based hierarchies. American Journal of Law and Medicine. 2017;**43**(2-3, 223):209. DOI: 10.1177/0098858817723660

[10] Hagiwara N, Lafata JE, Mezuk B, Vrana SR, Fetters MD. Detecting implicit racial bias in provider communication behaviors to reduce disparities in healthcare: Challenges, solutions, and future directions for provider communication training. Patient Education and Counseling. 2019;**102**(9):1738-1743. DOI: 10.1016/j.pec.2019.04.023

[11] Mabeza R. Reimagining medical education toward antiracist praxis. Health Equity. 2023;**7**(1):598-602. DOI: 10.1089/heq.2023.0135

[12] Hamed S, Bradby H, Ahlberg B, Thapar-Björkert S. Racism in healthcare: A scoping review. NYC: BMC Public Health. 2022;**22**(1):22. DOI: 10.1186/s12889-022-13122-y

[13] Matthew DB. Just Medicine: A Cure for Racial Inequality in American Health Care. New York: NYU Press; 2018. ISBN:978-1479851621

[14] Capers Q, Bond DA, Nori US. Bias and racism teaching rounds at an Academic Medical Center. Chest. 2020;**158**(6):2688-2694. DOI: 10.1016/j.chest.2020.08.2073

[15] Cerdeña JP, Asabor EN, Plaisime MV, Hardeman RR. Race-based medicine

in the point-of-care clinical resource UpToDate: A systematic content analysis. EClinicalMedicine. 2022;**52**:9. DOI: 10.1016/J.ECLINM.2022.101581

[16] Bakkum M. A clinical pharmacology and therapeutics teacher's guide to race-based medicine, inclusivity, and diversity. Clinical Pharmacology and Therapeutics. 2022;**113**(3):600-606. DOI: 10.1002/cpt.2786

[17] Bolnick D. Combating racial health disparities through medical education: The need for anthropological and genetic perspectives in medical training. Human Biology. 2015;**87**(4):361. DOI: 10.13110/humanbiology.87.4.0361

[18] Dent R, Vichare A, Casimir J. Addressing structural racism in the health workforce. Medical Care. 2021;**59**(Suppl. 5):S409-S412. DOI: 10.1097/mlr.0000000000001604

[19] Butts G. Designing a road map for action to address bias and racism within a large academic medical center. Academic Medicine. 2023;**98**(12):1381-1389. DOI: 10.1097/acm.0000000000005289

[20] Gruber J, Condon A. Does it work? Resident selection and implicit bias training for postgraduate program directors. Canadian Medical Education Journal. 2023;**14**(5):108-109. DOI: 10.36834/cmej.75861

[21] Elliott B. White Coat Ways: A History of Medical Traditions and their Battle with Progress. Med Media Publishing; 2023. ISBN 979-8218132217

[22] Roberts D. Fatal Invention: How Science, Politics, and Big Business Re-Create Race in the Twenty-First Century. The New Press; 2012. ISBN: 978-1595584953

[23] Bonham VL, Green ED, Pérez-Stable EJ. Examining how race, ethnicity, and ancestry data are used in biomedical research. JAMA. 2018;**320**(15):1533-1534. DOI: 10.1001/jama.2018.13609

[24] Schmeusser B, Palacios A, Midenberg E, Nabavizadeh R, Patil D, Harvey R, et al. Race-free renal function estimation equations and potential impact on black patients: Implications for cancer clinical trial enrollment. Cancer. 2023;**129**(6):920-924. DOI: 10.1002/cncr.34637

[25] Metzl JM, Hansen H. Structural competency: Theorizing a new medical engagement with stigma and inequality. Social Science and Medicine. 2014;**1982**(103):126-133. DOI: 10.1016/j.socscimed.2013.06.032

[26] Jubran N, Bratta P. Integrating institutional and individual self-reflexivity practices into clinical pharmacy practice: A critical review of race in a widely utilized medical guideline. Journal of the American College of Clinical Pharmacy. 2022;**5**(8):904-911. DOI: 10.1002/jac5.1665

[27] Pleasant V. The importance of discussing the history of racism in medical student education. Clinical Obstetrics and Gynecology. 2024;**67**(3):499-511. DOI: 10.1097/grf.0000000000000879

[28] Lai D, Lee V, Ruan Y. Perspectives towards cultural competence and receptivity to cultural competence training: A qualitative study on healthcare professionals. Primary Health Care Research and Development. 2023;**24**:8. DOI: 10.1017/s1463423623000245

[29] Hauer K, Park Y, Bullock J, Tekian A. "My assessments are biased!" measurement and sociocultural

approaches to achieve fairness in assessment in medical education. Academic Medicine. 2023;**98**(8S):S16-S27. DOI: 10.1097/acm.0000000000005245

[30] Lynn T, D'Urzo K, Vaughan-Ogunlusi O, Wiesendanger K, Colbert-Kaip S, Capcara A, et al. A student-led anti-racism program impacts medical students' perceptions and awareness of racial bias in medicine and confidence to advocate against racism. Medical Education Online. 2023;**28**(1):11. DOI: 10.1080/10872981.2023.2176802

[31] Denizard-Thompson N, Palakshappa D, Vallevand A, Kundu D, Brooks A, DiGiacobbe G, et al. Association of a health equity curriculum with medical students' knowledge of social determinants of health and confidence in working with underserved populations. JAMA Network Open. 2021;**4**(3):e210297. DOI: 10.1001/jamanetworkopen.2021.0297

[32] Vyas DA, Eisenstein LG, Jones DS. Hidden in plain sight-reconsidering the use of race correction in clinical algorithms. The New England Journal of Medicine. 2020;**383**(9):874-882. DOI: 10.1056/NEJMms2004740

[33] Williams DR, Cooper LA. Reducing racial inequities in health: Using what we already know to take action. International Journal of Environmental Research and Public Health. 2019;**16**(4):606. DOI: 10.3390/ijerph16040606

[34] Greilich P, Kilcullen M, Paquette S, Lazzara E, Scielzo S, Hernandez J, et al. Team first framework: Identifying core teamwork competencies critical to interprofessional healthcare curricula. Journal of. Clinical and Translational Science. 2023;**7**(1):7. DOI: 10.1017/cts.2023.27

[35] Li A, Deyrup A, Graves J, Ross L. Race in the reading: A study of problematic uses of race and ethnicity in a prominent pediatrics textbook. Academic Medicine. 2022;**97**(10):1521-1527. DOI: 10.1097/acm.0000000000004666

[36] Rollin F, Doren V, Alvarez J, Rousselle R, Bussey-Jones J. Antiracist structural intervention at the Emory University institutional review board. Ethics and Human Research. 2023;**45**(4):30-34. DOI: 10.1002/eahr.500174

[37] Tarleton C. Preparing Medical Students for Anti-Racism at the Bedside: Teaching Skills to Mitigate Racism and Bias in Clinical Encounters. Washington, DC: Mededportal; 2023. DOI: 10.15766/mep_2374-8265.11333

[38] Gravlee CC. How race becomes biology: Embodiment of social inequality. American Journal of Physical Anthropology. 2019;**139**(1):47-57. DOI: 10.1002/ajpa.20983

[39] Medicine IO, Policy B on HS, Care C on U and ER and ED in H. Unequal Treatment: Confronting Racial and Ethnic Disparities in Health Care. Washington, DC: National Academies Press; 2002. ISBN: 978-0309085328

[40] Mohottige D, Purnell T, Boulware L. Redressing the harms of race-based kidney function estimation. JAMA. 2023;**329**(11):881. DOI: 10.1001/jama.2023.2154

[41] Jones DD. Dismantling institutional racism: The role of behavioral science. The International Journal of Psychiatry in Medicine. 2022;**57**(5):373-380. DOI: 10.1177/00912174221111661

[42] Duffy TP. The Flexner report: 100 years later. International Journal

of Medical Education. 2010;**1**:74-75. DOI: 10.5116/ijme.4cb4.85c8

[43] Silver C, Williams S, Forty L. Cultural competency and mental health training for medical students: Learning from refugees and asylum seekers. Health Education Journal. 2023;**82**(6):708-721. DOI: 10.1177/00178969231182104

[44] Carrera D, Tejeda C, Kakani P, Napolitano J. Addressing racism in medical education: A longitudinal antiracism discussion curriculum for medical students. Medical Science Educator. 2023;**33**(3):639-643. DOI: 10.1007/s40670-023-01788-x

[45] Richmond S, Grubbs V. How abolition of race-based medicine is necessary to American health justice. The Ama Journal of Ethic. 2022;**24**(3):E226-E232. DOI: 10.1001/amajethics.2022.226

Chapter 6

Addressing Food Insecurity, Poverty, and Housing Insecurity in Medical Education: Integrating Social Determinants into Curriculum and Practice

Daryl O. Traylor and Eboni E. Anderson

Abstract

This chapter underscores the critical need to integrate social determinants of health (SDOH) into medical education, with a particular focus on food insecurity, poverty, and housing insecurity. These determinants profoundly impact health outcomes, perpetuate disparities, and place a significant burden on healthcare systems. By addressing these factors through targeted educational strategies, medical schools can prepare future physicians to identify, understand, and mitigate the systemic barriers to health equity. The chapter explores the multifaceted implications of these SDOH on physical and mental health, offering innovative educational strategies such as case-based learning, community partnerships, and interprofessional training to equip students with practical skills and empathy. It addresses the barriers to implementing SDOH-focused curricula, including time constraints and resistance from stakeholders, while highlighting opportunities such as advancements in virtual simulation technology and alignment with accreditation standards emphasizing health equity. Advocacy and institutional reforms are emphasized as pivotal components of equipping future physicians to champion systemic change and address health disparities. Ultimately, the chapter advocates for the integration of SDOH into medical education as a moral and practical imperative, fostering a healthcare workforce committed to advancing equitable health outcomes for all communities.

Keywords: social determinants of health, medical education, food insecurity, poverty, housing insecurity, health equity

1. Introduction

The social determinants of health (SDOH) encompass a range of environmental, economic, and social factors that profoundly influence individual and population health outcomes. Among these determinants, food insecurity, poverty, and housing instability stand out as critical issues that significantly impact health and exacerbate healthcare disparities [1]. These interconnected challenges restrict access to healthcare, undermine treatment efficacy, and perpetuate cycles of poor health. Addressing the SDOH is not simply about improving individual outcomes; it is foundational to achieving systemic health equity. By proactively integrating strategies to mitigate these challenges, healthcare systems can shift from reactive treatment to proactive health promotion, and foster resilience and equity for their patients.

Medical education plays a pivotal role in addressing these concerns, by equipping future physicians with the tools needed to identify and address the complexities of SDOH in both clinical and community settings. As awareness of the importance of SDOH grows, so does the demand for medical training that prepares physicians to navigate these pressing issues [2]. However, the integration of SDOH into medical curricula remains a challenging endeavor. Constraints such as limited instructional time, inadequate resources, and a lack of standardized teaching frameworks present significant barriers [3]. Overcoming these challenges is essential for cultivating a physician workforce capable of providing equitable care and advocating for systemic reforms to reduce disparities. Empowering future physicians with a deep understanding of SDOH will not only enhance patient care but also position physicians as leaders in broader societal efforts to advance health equity.

1.1 Overview of social determinants of health (SDOH)

1.1.1 Definitions and importance of food insecurity, poverty, and housing insecurity as critical SDOH

The term "social determinants of health" refers to the environmental, economic, and social conditions that shape the health and well-being of individuals and populations [4]. Food insecurity, poverty, and housing instability are among the most pressing SDOH, as they directly affect access to essential resources, influence health behaviors, and drive disparities in health outcomes [5]. These determinants are interlinked and create a cascade of challenges that not only hinder individual health but also place a burden on healthcare systems striving to achieve equitable care.

1.1.2 Relevance to patient outcomes and healthcare disparities

Food insecurity, poverty, and housing instability are closely tied to adverse health outcomes, including chronic diseases, mental health challenges, and reduced life expectancy [6]. Their effects extend beyond individual health, contributing to broader healthcare disparities and inequities within communities. Patients facing these determinants often experience delayed care, poorer adherence to treatment, and diminished overall health outcomes [7, 8]. These burdens are disproportionately felt by low-income individuals, women, children, and racial minorities, further exacerbating existing inequities [5]. These factors underscore the urgent need for healthcare systems and practitioners to address these factors holistically.

1.2 Role of medical education

1.2.1 The imperative to prepare future physicians to recognize and address these determinants

Future physicians must be equipped to identify and address the multifaceted impact of SDOH on patient health. Integrating SDOH into medical education will ensure that physicians understand the systemic nature of health disparities and will be prepared to adopt both clinical and advocacy roles to improve health equity. Recognizing and responding to SDOH is no longer a peripheral component of medical education but should be a core competency required for effective and compassionate patient care.

1.2.2 Challenges in integrating SDOH into medical curricula

Despite its importance, incorporating SDOH into medical curricula is fraught with challenges. Limited time within an already packed curriculum, resource constraints, and the absence of standardized frameworks for teaching these topics hinder progress [3]. Additionally, stakeholders may sometimes resist incorporating SDOH into medical school curricula and clinical practice due to a lack of understanding of its relevance [9]. Addressing these barriers is critical to fostering a physician workforce that is not only clinically proficient but also attuned to the social contexts that shape patient health.

1.2.3 Methodology

The methodology for this chapter was grounded in a thorough literature review. Sources were identified in academic databases, including PubMed, Google Scholar, JSTOR, Scopus, Web of Science, ProQuest, and ERIC, with a focus on terms such as "social determinants of health," "food insecurity," "poverty," "housing insecurity," "health equity," "medical education," "health disparities," "educational strategies," and "community-based interventions." Priority was given to peer-reviewed articles, gray literature, institutional guidelines, and textbooks to ensure relevance. Sources were selected based on their relevance to SDOH in medical education, their contribution to understanding health equity, and their methodological robustness, while those lacking empirical support or clear applicability were excluded.

2. Food insecurity

Food insecurity, as defined by the United States Department of Agriculture (USDA), is a condition in which households face uncertainty or inability to acquire sufficient food to meet the needs of all their members due to limited resources [10]. Food insecurity is a multifaceted issue that extends beyond simply having or lacking food. It encompasses three critical dimensions: food access, food availability, and food utilization [11]. Together, these dimensions highlight the systemic and structural factors underlying food insecurity, while underscoring its strong ties to the broader socioeconomic determinants of health. Addressing food insecurity requires a comprehensive understanding of these interconnected dimensions and the underlying barriers that perpetuate inequities. By tackling these challenges, we can create sustainable solutions that promote food equity and improve overall health outcomes.

Food access refers to the ability of individuals or households to obtain sufficient and nutritious food to sustain a healthy life [12]. This dimension is influenced by a variety of factors, including economic resources, proximity to food sources, and transportation infrastructure [13, 14]. For example, households in low-income neighborhoods often face challenges such as limited financial means and inadequate public transportation, making it difficult to reach stores that offer fresh, healthy, and affordable food. Without adequate food access, families may rely on inexpensive, calorie-dense foods that lack essential nutrients, perpetuating cycles of poor health.

Food availability highlights the adequacy of the food supply within a given region, addressing both the physical presence of food and the stability of its supply over time [15]. This dimension is shaped by factors such as agricultural productivity, market dynamics, and supply chain infrastructure [15]. In regions where food availability is compromised by economic disruptions, natural disasters, or political instability, communities may face challenges in accessing essential food items. This inconsistency further exacerbates food insecurity.

Food utilization focuses on how food is consumed and used to meet nutritional needs [12]. It encompasses dietary quality, food safety, and individuals' ability to derive maximum benefit from the food they consume [16]. Effective utilization requires not only the presence of nutritious food but also knowledge about its preparation and storage, as well as access to healthcare to address underlying health conditions that can impair nutrient absorption [16]. For instance, individuals with gastrointestinal disorders may have difficulty absorbing nutrients even when their food intake appears sufficient. This emphasizes the importance of addressing food utilization as a critical dimension of food insecurity.

Together, these dimensions illustrate that food insecurity extends far beyond a simple lack of food, reflecting deep-seated structural inequities and socioeconomic disparities. By understanding food insecurity through the lens of access, availability, and utilization, we can begin to address its root causes and develop interventions that promote equity and health in vulnerable populations. Addressing these interconnected factors requires coordinated efforts at the individual, community, and policy levels to ensure sustainable solutions. Only through such comprehensive approaches can we hope to break the cycle of food insecurity and build healthier, more resilient communities for future generations.

2.1 Health implications

Food insecurity has profound implications for physical, mental, and social well-being. Nutritional deficiencies, resulting from limited access to a diverse and balanced diet, are a primary concern. These deficiencies are associated with a heightened risk of chronic diseases such as diabetes, hypertension, and obesity, as individuals often rely on inexpensive, calorie-dense, but nutritionally poor foods [17].

The consequences extend beyond physical health. Food insecurity is a significant predictor of poor mental health outcomes, including depression, anxiety, and stress [18]. For children, it has been linked to developmental delays, cognitive impairments, and behavioral issues, further perpetuating cycles of disadvantage [19]. Adults experiencing food insecurity are more likely to report feelings of isolation and diminished quality of life, highlighting the pervasive impact of inadequate access to food on overall health and well-being [20].

2.1.1 Educational strategies

To effectively address food insecurity in medical education, innovative and practical strategies are essential. These approaches should not only enhance students' understanding of the issue but also prepare future physicians to identify and mitigate food insecurity in their practice. By embedding real-world applications and collaborative experiences into the curriculum, educators can cultivate a deeper comprehension of this critical public health challenge.

One effective strategy is the use of case-based learning, which incorporates patient scenarios that highlight the complexities of food insecurity [21]. These scenarios provide students with a platform to apply theoretical knowledge to realistic contexts. For instance, students might analyze cases involving patients managing chronic diseases exacerbated by inadequate nutrition or families navigating limited resources to access healthy foods. Through guided discussions, they learn to identify food insecurity as a determinant of health and explore patient-centered interventions, fostering critical thinking and practical problem-solving skills.

Another possible approach involves collaboration with community organizations. Partnerships with local food banks, community gardens, and nonprofit organizations offer students valuable experiential learning opportunities [22, 23]. Engaging in food distribution, nutrition education programs, or community advocacy initiatives enables students to observe firsthand the challenges and nuances of addressing food insecurity. These experiences emphasize the importance of collaborative, community-based solutions and highlight the role of social determinants of health in shaping outcomes.

Training in the use of screening tools and interventions further equips students to address food insecurity effectively [24]. Familiarity with validated tools such as the Hunger Vital Sign enables future professionals to identify food insecurity in both clinical and community settings [25, 26]. These tools facilitate early recognition and prompt interventions, allowing professionals to connect individuals and families with appropriate resources [26]. Additionally, integrating training on interventions—including referrals to food assistance programs, nutrition counseling, and policy advocacy—ensures that students are prepared to address food insecurity holistically and sustainably.

By integrating case-based learning, community collaboration, and training in screening tools and interventions into educational curricula, educators can empower students to address food insecurity with sensitivity, creativity, and practical expertise. These strategies not only enhance professional readiness but also foster a generation of public health and healthcare practitioners committed to improving food equity and advancing health outcomes in the communities they serve.

3. Poverty

3.1 Understanding poverty

Poverty is a multifaceted social determinant of health, defined by a lack of financial resources to meet basic needs, including housing, food, healthcare, and education [27]. Frameworks for defining and measuring poverty often utilize absolute and relative thresholds. Absolute poverty measures focus on income levels necessary to sustain minimal living standards, such as the federal poverty line in the United States [28].

Relative poverty measures compare individuals' economic status to the median income within their society, highlighting inequalities that contribute to social exclusion [28].

The relationship between poverty and health is complex and multifaceted. Economic deprivation limits access to nutritious food, stable housing, and healthcare, resulting in poorer health outcomes. In turn, health issues can reduce earning potential, further entrenching individuals in poverty [29]. This cycle disproportionately affects marginalized populations, amplifying disparities and perpetuating generational inequities.

3.2 Clinical impact of poverty

Poverty significantly impacts clinical outcomes through delayed healthcare access, poor treatment adherence, and disparities in health outcomes. Financial barriers often deter individuals from seeking timely medical care, leading to advanced disease stages at diagnosis and increased morbidity [30]. Similarly, the costs associated with transportation, medication, and follow-up appointments exacerbate treatment non-adherence, particularly for chronic conditions like diabetes or hypertension [31].

Disparities in outcomes are also evident across populations. Individuals experiencing poverty are at heightened risk for preventable hospitalizations and worse prognoses compared to those with higher incomes [32]. These challenges underscore the necessity for healthcare providers to address poverty-related barriers as part of comprehensive patient care.

3.2.1 Educational approaches to teaching medical students about poverty

Preparing medical students to address poverty as a social determinant of health requires an integrative approach to education. Curricula must emphasize practical skills and empathy to navigate healthcare systems for underserved populations. Key educational strategies include:

- *Navigating healthcare systems for underserved populations*

  Students should learn to identify systemic barriers and facilitate access to care for economically disadvantaged patients. This includes training in referral pathways for social services, financial assistance programs, and community-based health resources.

- *Simulations to understand economic constraints*

  Simulated activities, such as budgeting exercises or patient case scenarios, help students grasp the constraints faced by patients living in poverty. These exercises illustrate the trade-offs individuals must make between healthcare and other necessities, fostering empathy and systems-thinking.

- *Advocacy training to address systemic barriers*

  Advocacy education equips future physicians to champion policies that reduce poverty-related health disparities. Through workshops and experiential learning, students gain skills in legislative advocacy, community engagement, and interprofessional collaboration.

By integrating these approaches, medical education can cultivate physicians who are not only clinically competent but also attuned to the broader social and economic contexts shaping patient health.

4. Housing insecurity

4.1 Scope and impact of housing insecurity

Housing insecurity encompasses a spectrum of challenges, ranging from homelessness to frequent relocations and substandard living environments [33]. Homelessness, as defined by the U.S. Department of Housing and Urban Development, refers to the lack of a fixed, regular, and adequate nighttime residence [34]. This includes individuals living in shelters, transitional housing, or public spaces. Unstable housing often manifests as overcrowded living conditions, precarious lease agreements, or the inability to afford housing costs consistently. These situations reflect broader systemic inequities in economic stability, access to affordable housing, and social support.

Housing insecurity has profound implications for physical and mental health. Substandard living conditions expose individuals to hazards such as mold, lead, and pests, contributing to respiratory issues, chronic illnesses, and increased risk of infections [35]. Overcrowding facilitates the spread of communicable diseases, while the stress of unstable housing exacerbates mental health conditions, including anxiety, depression, and post-traumatic stress disorder. Children experiencing housing insecurity are particularly vulnerable, with evidence linking it to developmental delays, behavioral issues, and academic underachievement [36]. These outcomes underline the critical intersection of housing and health.

4.2 Clinical considerations

Overcrowding, a common feature of housing insecurity, amplifies the risk of communicable diseases such as tuberculosis and influenza [37]. Substandard housing often lacks adequate ventilation, heating, or sanitation, exposing occupants to environmental toxins and exacerbating chronic conditions like asthma. For individuals experiencing homelessness, the lack of access to clean water, nutritious food, and healthcare services increases susceptibility to injuries, untreated medical conditions, and exposure-related health issues such as hypothermia. Clinicians must be prepared to address these interconnected risks with targeted interventions and resource referrals.

4.3 Incorporating housing insecurity into community medicine rotations

Community medicine rotations can offer medical students' invaluable insights into housing insecurity [38, 39]. By engaging directly with affected populations, students develop practical skills in assessing housing-related health risks and connecting patients to social and medical resources [39]. These rotations also encourage a holistic approach to patient care, emphasizing the importance of addressing environmental and social determinants alongside clinical treatment.

Collaborations with housing organizations enable students to participate in multidisciplinary care, combining medical treatment with housing assistance [40].

For example, partnerships with shelters or transitional housing programs can provide opportunities for students to learn about comprehensive care models that address both health and housing needs.

Storytelling and patient narratives are powerful tools for fostering empathy among medical students [41]. By hearing firsthand accounts of individuals navigating housing insecurity, students gain a deeper understanding of the systemic barriers and personal struggles involved [42]. These narratives help future physicians approach patient care with greater sensitivity and awareness of the broader social context.

5. Integrating SDOH into medical curricula

5.1 Frameworks for embedding SDOH in pre-clinical and clinical phases

To ensure a comprehensive understanding of social determinants of health (SDOH), medical education must adopt a structured, longitudinal approach spanning pre-clinical and clinical training phases. In the pre-clinical phase, foundational concepts of SDOH can be introduced through a combination of lectures, interactive seminars, and case-based learning modules. For example, students might analyze patient scenarios illustrating how SDOH influence clinical decision-making, such as a case involving a patient with poor diabetes control due to food insecurity. Small group discussions and reflective exercises can further solidify their theoretical understanding.

The clinical phase should emphasize experiential learning, with students applying SDOH principles in real-world contexts. Rotations in underserved or rural communities provide invaluable opportunities to witness firsthand the barriers patients face in accessing healthcare [43]. These rotations can include tasks like conducting home visits, participating in community health outreach, or working in free clinics. Through this phased approach, students not only acquire knowledge about SDOH but also develop the skills needed to address these challenges in practice.

Addressing SDOH requires collaboration among diverse professionals, making interprofessional education (IPE) a critical component of medical training. Effective IPE programs teach students to work alongside social workers, case managers, public health professionals, and community health workers [44]. Such training highlights the complementary roles of these stakeholders in mitigating SDOH-related barriers to care. For instance, social workers can assist with housing stability, while case managers help patients navigate healthcare systems to access needed services.

Simulation exercises that replicate multidisciplinary team meetings or interprofessional case conferences can prepare students for collaborative practice. These activities foster mutual respect and understanding of each professional's contributions to patient care, emphasizing that addressing SDOH is a shared responsibility.

5.2 Measuring student competency in identifying and addressing SDOH

Assessment is crucial for ensuring that students not only understand SDOH conceptually but can also apply this knowledge effectively in clinical settings. One effective tool is the use of Objective Structured Clinical Examinations (OSCEs), where students interact with standardized patients presenting with SDOH-related challenges. For instance, an OSCE station might involve a patient who is unable to adhere to medication due to financial constraints, requiring the student to identify the barrier and propose appropriate interventions [45].

Reflective essays and portfolios also serve as valuable assessment methods [43]. These assignments allow students to analyze their experiences addressing SDOH during clinical rotations or community projects, offering insights into their growth and understanding.

To ensure sustained competency, longitudinal evaluation mechanisms should track students' ability to address SDOH throughout their education and into residency. Tools such as 360-degree feedback—where peers, faculty, and patients provide input—can help assess students' interpersonal and problem-solving skills [46]. Additionally, periodic evaluations, including case presentations that highlight SDOH interventions, ensure that graduates remain adept at integrating these principles into their clinical practice. Long-term tracking can also assess the impact of SDOH education on healthcare outcomes and patient satisfaction.

5.3 Faculty development and resources for teaching SDOH

Faculty are central to successfully integrating SDOH into medical curricula, yet many lack the training or resources to effectively teach these concepts. Institutions should invest in faculty development through workshops, mentorship programs, and access to teaching materials [47, 48]. For instance, seminars on using case-based learning to teach SDOH or strategies for integrating community partnerships into rotations can enhance faculty preparedness. Additionally, providing access to teaching aids, such as pre-designed case scenarios or SDOH-focused assessment tools, reduces the burden on faculty and promotes consistency across courses.

Accreditation standards increasingly emphasize the importance of addressing health disparities, creating an opportunity to align SDOH education with institutional priorities. For example, the Liaison Committee on Medical Education (LCME) requires that medical schools prepare students to address the health needs of underserved populations [49]. Aligning SDOH curricula with these requirements ensures institutional support and accountability. Additionally, integrating SDOH into the mission statements of medical schools reinforces the importance of health equity and encourages sustained investment in these programs [46]. Schools can further promote this alignment by showcasing their SDOH initiatives in annual reports and accreditation documents, demonstrating their commitment to addressing disparities.

6. Best practices and case studies

6.1 Analysis of medical schools successfully integrating food insecurity, poverty, and housing insecurity topics

Across the United States, several medical schools have emerged as leaders in integrating social determinants of health (SDOH) into their curricula, particularly focusing on food insecurity, poverty, and housing instability [50–55]. These schools often adopt innovative, community-oriented strategies that extend beyond traditional didactic teaching. For instance, the University of Texas Southwestern School of Medicine (UTSW) incorporates community-based participatory research (CBPR) into its curriculum [56]. Through CBPR, students collaborate with local organizations to identify community health needs, develop interventions, and evaluate their impact. This model not only reinforces academic learning but also fosters a deeper connection between students and the communities they serve.

Similarly, at Morehouse School of Medicine, students participate in initiatives that directly address housing insecurity [56]. The curriculum includes fieldwork in community shelters and public housing projects, allowing students to observe the health impacts of unstable housing firsthand. By combining classroom learning with experiential opportunities, these programs ensure students understand both the theoretical and practical aspects of addressing SDOH. Moreover, these programs often result in tangible health benefits for underserved populations, such as improved disease management and increased access to preventive care services [57].

Mobile clinics have proven to be an exceptional innovation for integrating SDOH into medical education. For example, Harvard Medical School's Family Van program serves as a model for mobile healthcare delivery [58]. This program not only provides essential health services to low-income neighborhoods but also offers students hands-on experience with patient care in resource-limited settings. Students are actively involved in conducting health screenings, counseling patients, and referring them to community resources, fostering a comprehensive understanding of the barriers patients face.

Community outreach programs, such as those run by the University of Michigan, similarly prepare students to address SDOH by engaging them in partnerships with food banks, housing advocacy groups, and public health departments [59]. These initiatives often include health fairs, where students provide free health services and education to residents. By working directly with underserved populations, students learn to navigate complex systems of care, build cultural competency, and develop empathy for patients experiencing food and housing insecurity.

6.2 Lessons learned

Despite the success of these programs, implementing SDOH-focused curricula is not without challenges. One significant obstacle is the limited time available in already dense medical school schedules. Balancing foundational science courses with new SDOH content requires strategic curriculum design to ensure essential topics are covered without overburdening students. Additionally, resource constraints—such as limited funding for community partnerships or inadequate faculty training—can hinder program development. Faculty resistance can also present a barrier, particularly when instructors are unfamiliar with SDOH topics or skeptical about their relevance to clinical practice. Overcoming these hurdles demands institutional commitment to prioritizing SDOH education.

To ensure sustainability, programs must secure long-term funding through grants, partnerships with healthcare organizations, or institutional budgets. For example, many successful initiatives, such as the mobile clinics at Johns Hopkins University, rely on funding from local healthcare systems and philanthropic donations [60]. Additionally, fostering strong community partnerships is critical. Engaging local stakeholders, such as housing organizations and food banks, creates mutually beneficial relationships that enhance program impact and longevity.

Scaling successful interventions requires sharing best practices across institutions. Conferences, journal publications, and online forums can facilitate this exchange of ideas. Furthermore, adapting proven models to fit the unique contexts of different medical schools is essential. For instance, a mobile clinic program developed in an urban setting may need modifications to address the specific challenges of rural healthcare delivery. By promoting adaptability and collaboration, medical schools can ensure that effective SDOH initiatives are implemented widely, improving health equity on a broader scale.

7. Barriers and opportunities

7.1 Barriers

Medical education is notoriously rigorous, with a dense curriculum that spans foundational sciences, clinical skills, and specialty training. Adding comprehensive SDOH content to this already packed schedule is a significant challenge. Educators often struggle to balance the inclusion of new material with existing requirements, particularly given the constraints imposed by standardized exams such as the United States Medical Licensing Examination (USMLE) and Comprehensive Osteopathic Medical Licensing Examination (COMLEX) [61]. Without careful planning and prioritization, SDOH topics risk being treated as peripheral rather than integral components of medical training.

To address this barrier, curriculum committees must identify opportunities for integration rather than supplementation. For example, SDOH concepts can be woven into existing courses such as pathology or pharmacology by emphasizing case studies that highlight the interplay between social determinants and disease progression. Another approach is to embed SDOH within clinical skills training, using patient scenarios that require students to identify and address factors such as housing instability or food insecurity [57, 62]. By leveraging these strategies, schools can ensure that SDOH education is seamlessly incorporated without overwhelming students or compromising core content.

Another significant barrier is resistance from stakeholders, including faculty, administrators, and policymakers, who may question the relevance of SDOH in medical education [3]. This skepticism often stems from a lack of awareness about the profound impact of social determinants on health outcomes. Some stakeholders may view SDOH as tangential to the biomedical focus of medical training, arguing that these topics are better suited for public health programs or social work.

Overcoming this resistance requires advocacy and the use of evidence-based arguments. Educators and proponents of SDOH integration should highlight compelling data demonstrating the links between social determinants and health outcomes. For instance, studies consistently show that addressing SDOH can reduce hospital readmissions, improve chronic disease management, and lower healthcare costs. Engaging stakeholders in workshops, seminars, or panel discussions with clinicians who have successfully incorporated SDOH into practice can also help bridge this gap in understanding. By demonstrating the practical value of SDOH education, advocates can foster buy-in and promote cultural change within institutions.

7.2 Opportunities

Recent shifts in medical education and public health policy have created a favorable climate for integrating SDOH into medical education [60]. Accreditation bodies such as the LCME and the Accreditation Council for Graduate Medical Education (ACGME) now emphasize the importance of health equity and community engagement. For example, the LCME's standards include requirements for teaching students to identify and address health disparities, providing a framework for embedding SDOH into curricula [2].

Public health mandates further bolster this momentum. Agencies like the Centers for Disease Control and Prevention (CDC) and the World Health Organization

(WHO) have prioritized social determinants as critical to achieving population health goals [63]. This alignment with broader societal objectives allows medical schools to position SDOH education as not only a curricular innovation but also a moral and institutional imperative. Schools can leverage these mandates to secure funding, build faculty capacity, and justify curricular reforms.

Community partnerships offer rich opportunities for enhancing SDOH education. Collaborating with organizations such as food banks, housing advocacy groups, and public health departments allows students to engage directly with underserved populations, providing experiential learning that complements classroom instruction. These partnerships also create opportunities for service-learning projects, community-based participatory research, and interprofessional training, ensuring students gain practical skills in addressing social determinants.

Advances in technology provide additional avenues for innovation. Virtual simulations, for instance, enable students to explore SDOH-related scenarios in a controlled, immersive environment [64]. These patient simulations can replicate the challenges faced by patients with limited financial resources or unstable housing. These tools allow students to practice problem-solving, develop empathy, and refine their clinical decision-making without the logistical constraints of traditional fieldwork. By combining technological innovations with community-based initiatives, medical schools can scale SDOH education effectively, reaching more students and maximizing impact.

8. Policy and advocacy

8.1 Training students to engage in policy discussions at local, state, and national levels

Physicians have a unique and powerful role in advocating for systemic changes that address SDOH. To prepare students for this role, medical education must include structured training in policy advocacy. This training should emphasize the intersection of healthcare and public policy, equipping future physicians with the skills needed to engage in meaningful dialog with policymakers at various levels.

Practical exercises can significantly enhance students' advocacy skills. For instance, workshops on drafting policy briefs allow students to synthesize evidence and articulate actionable recommendations tailored to local, state, or national contexts. These briefs can address pressing issues such as expanding Medicaid coverage, funding affordable housing programs, or supporting food assistance initiatives. Additionally, organizing advocacy days, where students meet with legislators to discuss health equity concerns, offers real-world experience in influencing policy decisions. By exposing students to these activities during their training, medical schools can cultivate a generation of physicians who are not only clinical experts but also effective advocates for systemic change.

Moreover, role-playing scenarios in educational settings can simulate policy debates, helping students anticipate counterarguments and refine their messaging. Encouraging participation in professional organizations, such as the American Medical Association (AMA) or local medical societies, further empowers students to engage in policy advocacy and amplify their voices within larger healthcare movements [65].

DOI: http://dx.doi.org/10.5772/intechopen.1009497

8.2 Collaborating with stakeholders

Collaboration with public health agencies, non-profit organizations, and government programs is essential for amplifying the impact of advocacy efforts. These partnerships enable physicians and medical students to address systemic barriers to health equity more effectively by pooling resources, expertise, and networks.

Public health agencies, such as local health departments or the CDC, provide valuable data and research that inform evidence-based advocacy. For example, partnering with health departments allows students to understand regional disparities in housing, food security, or healthcare access, creating a foundation for targeted policy initiatives. Non-profits, such as Habitat for Humanity or Feeding America, bring on-the-ground experience and community trust, making them ideal collaborators for outreach and intervention programs [66].

Government programs, including Medicaid and the Supplemental Nutrition Assistance Program (SNAP), are critical levers for addressing SDOH [67]. Medical students can participate in initiatives that advocate for the expansion or preservation of these programs. For instance, engaging in campaigns to prevent funding cuts or improve program accessibility fosters an understanding of the intricate relationship between policy decisions and patient outcomes.

Collaborative partnerships also present opportunities for service-learning. By working alongside these stakeholders, students gain practical insights into the systemic nature of health inequities and learn how multi-sectoral collaboration can drive change. These experiences prepare them to navigate complex policy environments and advocate for sustainable solutions.

8.3 Institutional change

Healthcare institutions play a pivotal role in addressing SDOH and advancing health equity. By adopting policies and practices that prioritize SDOH, institutions can lead by example, influencing the broader healthcare landscape and reinforcing the importance of advocacy in medical practice.

One way institutions can act is by integrating SDOH considerations into patient care protocols. For example, hospitals and clinics can implement routine screening for food insecurity, housing instability, and transportation barriers as part of the intake process. These screenings enable early identification of needs and facilitate referrals to community resources or in-house support programs, such as social work services or care coordination teams.

Institutions should also invest in community outreach initiatives that address the root causes of health disparities. Collaborating with local organizations to establish free clinics, mobile health units, or housing assistance programs demonstrates a commitment to tackling SDOH beyond the clinical setting. These efforts not only improve community health outcomes but also create opportunities for medical students to witness the impact of SDOH interventions firsthand.

From a policy perspective, healthcare institutions should advocate for systemic reforms at the local, state, and national levels. By aligning institutional goals with advocacy efforts, hospitals and academic medical centers can leverage their influence to drive legislative change. For example, endorsing policies that fund affordable housing or expand public transportation access can directly benefit the patient populations they serve.

Finally, institutions must ensure their internal policies reflect a commitment to equity. This includes offering continuing education on SDOH for staff, hiring diverse leadership teams, and addressing workplace disparities. By fostering an organizational culture that prioritizes health equity, healthcare institutions can serve as role models for the medical community and beyond.

9. Conclusions

This chapter underscores the critical need to integrate food insecurity, poverty, and housing insecurity into medical education as essential SDOH. These interconnected challenges profoundly impact individual and population health, perpetuating disparities and placing a significant burden on healthcare systems. By addressing these determinants through targeted educational strategies, medical schools can prepare future physicians to identify, understand, and mitigate the systemic barriers to health equity.

The chapter explored the multifaceted nature of food insecurity, poverty, and housing insecurity, detailing their implications for physical and mental health. It emphasized the importance of equipping students with clinical and advocacy skills to navigate these issues effectively. Incorporating SDOH into pre-clinical and clinical training was presented as a transformative approach, fostering both theoretical knowledge and practical application. Examples of exemplary programs, such as mobile clinics and community outreach initiatives, showcased innovative methods for bridging the gap between medical education and real-world challenges.

Additionally, the chapter addressed the barriers to implementing SDOH-focused curricula, including time constraints and resistance from stakeholders. These challenges were counterbalanced by emerging opportunities, such as increased emphasis on health equity in accreditation standards and advancements in educational technology, like virtual simulations. Collaboration with public health agencies, non-profits, and government programs further highlighted the importance of partnerships in driving sustainable change.

The role of physicians as advocates was also explored, emphasizing the need for medical students to engage in policy discussions and institutional reforms that prioritize SDOH. By fostering interprofessional collaboration and promoting institutional practices that address health disparities, healthcare systems can lead by example, creating a culture of equity and compassion.

In conclusion, integrating SDOH into medical education is not merely an academic exercise but a moral and practical imperative. As future physicians, medical students must be equipped to address the root causes of health disparities, champion equity in healthcare, and advocate for systemic change. By embracing this vision, medical education can cultivate a generation of healthcare professionals committed to advancing health equity and improving outcomes for all communities.

Conflict of interest

The authors declare no conflict of interest.

Author details

Daryl O. Traylor[1*] and Eboni E. Anderson[2]

1 Eastern Washington University, Spokane, WA, United States

2 A.T. Still University School of Osteopathic Medicine at Arizona, Mesa, AZ, United States

*Address all correspondence to: dtraylor1@ewu.edu

References

[1] Daniel H, Bornstein SS, Kane GC, Health and Public Policy Committee of the American College of Physicians. Addressing social determinants to improve patient care and promote health equity: An American College of Physicians Position Paper. Annals of Internal Medicine. 2018;**168**(8):577-578. DOI: 10.7326/M17-2441

[2] Sandhu S, Solomon L, Gottlieb LM. Awareness, adjustment, assistance, alignment, and advocacy: Operationalizing social determinants of health topics in undergraduate medical education curricula. Academic Medicine. 2023;**98**(8):876-881. DOI: 10.1097/ACM.0000000000005223

[3] Lewis JH, Lage OG, Grant BK, Rajasekaran SK, Gemeda M, Like RC, et al. Addressing the social determinants of health in undergraduate medical education curricula: A survey report. Advances in Medical Education and Practice. 2020;**11**:369-377. DOI: 10.2147/AMEP.S243827

[4] Lipman TH, Lobo ML. Special issue on social determinants of health. Journal of Pediatric Nursing. 2017;**37**:1-2. DOI: 10.1016/j.pedn.2017.09.004. Epub 2017 Oct 6

[5] Bonnell LN, Crocker AM, Kemp K, Littenberg B. The relationship between social determinants of health and functional capacity in adult primary care patients with multiple chronic conditions. Journal of American Board of Family Medicine. 2021;**34**(4):688-697. DOI: 10.3122/jabfm.2021.04.210010

[6] Parekh T, Xue H, Cheskin LJ, Cuellar AE. Food insecurity and housing instability as determinants of cardiovascular health outcomes: A systematic review. Nutrition, Metabolism, and Cardiovascular Diseases. 2022;**32**(7):1590-1608. DOI: 10.1016/j.numecd.2022.03.025

[7] Ma CT, Gee L, Kushel MB. Associations between housing instability and food insecurity with health care access in low-income children. Ambulatory Pediatrics. 2008;**8**(1):50-57. DOI: 10.1016/j.ambp.2007.08.004

[8] Kushel MB, Gupta R, Gee L, Haas JS. Housing instability and food insecurity as barriers to health care among low-income Americans. Journal of General Internal Medicine. 2006;**21**:71-77. DOI: 10.1111/j.1525-1497.2005.00278.x

[9] Petrin C, DeSalvo K. Moving upstream to impact health: Building a physician workforce that understands social determinants. North Carolina Medical Journal. 2020;**81**(3):188-191. DOI: 10.18043/ncm.81.3.188

[10] Castillo DC, Ramsey NLM, Yu SSK, et al. Inconsistent access to food and cardiometabolic disease: The effect of food insecurity. Current Cardiovascular Risk Reports. 2012;**6**:245-250. DOI: 10.1007/s12170-012-0236-2

[11] Opara UL. Perspective: The evolving dimensions and perspectives on food security—What are the implications for postharvest technology research, policy and practice? International Journal of Postharvest Technology and Innovation. 2014;**3**(3):324-332. DOI: 10.1504/IJPTI.2013.059340

[12] Stifel D, Hassen IW. Food security. Africa Research Bulletin: Economic, Financial and Technical Series. 2020;**56**(12):22824B-22824D. DOI: 10.1111/j.1467-6346.2020.09291.x

[13] Tach L, Amorim M. Constrained, convenient, and symbolic consumption: Neighborhood food environments and economic coping strategies among the urban poor. Journal of Urban Health. 2015;**92**(5):815-834. DOI: 10.1007/s11524-015-9984-x

[14] Vivian EM, Le J, Ikem P, Tolson Y. Health needs and neighbourhood concerns of low-income households vulnerable to food insecurity. Public Health. 2014;**128**(8):743-745. DOI: 10.1016/j.puhe.2014.05.005

[15] Hwalla N, El Labban S, Bahn RA. Nutrition security is an integral component of food security. Frontiers in Life Science. 2016;**9**(3):167-172. DOI: 10.1080/21553769.2016.1209133

[16] EC—FAO Food Security Programme. An Introduction to the Basic Concepts of Food Security. Rome: Food and Agriculture Organization; 2008. Available from: http://www.foodsec.org/docs/concepts_guide.pdf

[17] Thomas MK, Lammert LJ, Beverly EA. Food insecurity and its impact on body weight, type 2 diabetes, cardiovascular disease, and mental health. Current Cardiovascular Risk Reports. 2021;**15**:15. DOI: 10.1007/s12170-021-00679-3

[18] Martin MS, Maddocks E, Chen Y, Gilman SE, Colman I. Food insecurity and mental illness: Disproportionate impacts in the context of perceived stress and social isolation. Public Health. 2016;**132**:86-91. DOI: 10.1016/j.puhe.2015.11.014

[19] Collins L. The impact of food insecurity on women's mental health: How it negatively affects children's health and development. Journal of the Association for Research on Mothering. 2009;**11**(1):251-262. Available from: https://www.fao.org/docs/concepts_guide.pdf

[20] Cain KS, Meyer SC, Cummer E, Patel KK, Casacchia NJ, Montez K, et al. Association of food insecurity with mental health outcomes in parents and children. Academic Pediatrics. 2022;**22**(7):1105-1114. DOI: 10.1016/j.acap.2022.04.010

[21] Brown BD, Haley SP, Berini CR, Ramsetty AN. A novel case-based learning activity with a focus on food insecurity. Journal of Medical Education and Curricular Development. 2023;**10**:1-5. DOI: 10.1177/232123672312367

[22] Palakshappa D, Denizard-Thompson N, Puccinelli-Ortega N, Brooks A, Damman A, Miller DP Jr. The experiences of community organizations partnering with a medical school to improve students' understanding of the social determinants of health: A qualitative study. Medical Teacher. 2022;**44**(11):1260-1267. DOI: 10.1080/0142159X.2022.2056007

[23] O'Brien MJ, Garland JM, Murphy KM, Shuman SJ, Whitaker RC, Larson SC. Training medical students in the social determinants of health: The Health Scholars Program at Puentes de Salud. Advances in Medical Education and Practice. 2014;**5**:307-314. DOI: 10.2147/AMEP.S67480

[24] Jarris YS, Chang H, Kureshi S, Mishori R, Kaljee L, Hunting J, et al. Screening for food insecurity: A curriculum for medical students. PRiMER. 2024;**8**:9. DOI: 10.22454/PRiMER.2024.858771

[25] Nanaimo Foodshare Society. Hunger Vital Sign Screening Tool. Nanaimo: Nanaimo Foodshare Society; 2020. Available from: https://nanaimofoodshare.ca/wp-content/

uploads/2020/12/Hunger-Vital-Sign-Screening-Tool.pdf

[26] Stenmark SH, Steiner JF, Marpadga S, Debor M, Underhill K, Seligman H. Lessons learned from implementation of the Food Insecurity Screening and Referral Program at Kaiser Permanente Colorado. The Permanente Journal. 2018;**22**:18-093. DOI: 10.7812/TPP/18-093

[27] McCally M, Haines A, Fein O, Addington W, Lawrence RS, Cassel CK. Poverty and ill health: Physicians can, and should, make a difference. Annals of Internal Medicine. 1998;**129**(9):726-733. DOI: 10.7326/0003-4819-129-9-199811010-00009

[28] Cauthen NK, Fass S. Measuring Income and Poverty in the United States. New York (NY): National Center for Children in Poverty, Mailman School of Public Health, Columbia University; 2008. Available from: http://www.nccp.org

[29] Mukherjee K. Poverty as a cause and consequence of ill health. International Journal of Epidemiologic Research. 2015;**2**:209-220. Available from: https://typeset.io/pdf/poverty-as-a-cause-and-consequence-of-ill-health-2tm9szpn5w.pdf

[30] Campbell DJT, Manns BJ, Weaver RG, et al. Financial barriers and adverse clinical outcomes among patients with cardiovascular-related chronic diseases: A cohort study. BMC Medicine. 2017;**15**:33. DOI: 10.1186/s12916-017-0788-6

[31] Syed ST, Gerber BS, Sharp LK. Traveling towards disease: Transportation barriers to health care access. Journal of Community Health. 2013;**38**:976-993. DOI: 10.1007/s10900-013-9681-1

[32] Andrulis DP. Access to care is the centerpiece in the elimination of socioeconomic disparities in health. Annals of Internal Medicine. 1998;**129**(5):412-416. DOI: 10.7326/0003-4819-129-5-199809010-00012

[33] Hallett RE, Crutchfield R. Homelessness and housing insecurity in higher education: A trauma-informed approach to research, policy, and practice. AEHE. 2017;**43**(6):7-118. DOI: 10.1002/aehe.20122

[34] Swick KJ. The dynamics of families who are homeless: Implications for early childhood educators. Childhood Education. 2004;**80**(3):116-121. DOI: 10.1080/00094056.2004.10522786

[35] Bhat A, Almeida D, Santos A. Post-recession housing insecurity and physical and mental health of midlife and aging adults. Innovation in Aging. 2021;**5**(Suppl. 1):777. DOI: 10.1093/geroni/igab046.2873

[36] Bess KD, Miller AL, Mehdipanah R. The effects of housing insecurity on children's health: A scoping review. Health Promotion International. 2023;**38**(3):daac006. DOI: 10.1093/heapro/daac006

[37] Moffa M, Cronk R, Fejfar D, Dancausse S, Acosta Padilla L, Bartram J. A systematic scoping review of environmental health conditions and hygiene behaviors in homeless shelters. International Journal of Hygiene and Environmental Health. 2019;**222**(3):335-346. DOI: 10.1016/j.ijheh.2018.12.004

[38] Burke K, Bigham G, Ferrara-Leach G. A case-based workshop training medical students in assessing social determinants of health needs and connecting with community resources. MedEdPORTAL. 2022;**18**:11232. DOI: 10.15766/mep_2374-8265.11232

[39] Kangovi S, Carter T, Smith RA, DeLisser HM. A community health

worker-led rotation to train medical students in the social determinants of health. Journal of Health Care for the Poor and Underserved. 2018;**29**(2):581-590. DOI: 10.1353/hpu.2018.0042

[40] Dubbaka S, Lentz T. The importance of understanding social determinants of health as medical students: My experience with the Cincinnati Homeless Coalition. International Journal of Medical Students. 2022;**12**(1):109-111. DOI: 10.5195/ijms.2022.215

[41] Pattanaik D, Purvis E, Jeffrey D. Storytelling: A learning tool to enhance medical students' empathy, attentive listening, clinical curiosity and reflection. The Journal of the Royal College of Physicians of Edinburgh. 2024;**54**(4):325-329. DOI: 10.1177/14782715241299839

[42] Player E, Gure-Klinke H, North S, Hanson S, Lane D, Culyer G. Humanising medicine: Teaching on tri-morbidity using expert patient narratives in medical education. Education for Primary Care. 2019;**30**(6):368-374. DOI: 10.1080/14739879.2019.1670097

[43] Nielsen M, D'Agostino D, Gregory P. Addressing rural health challenges head on. Missouri Medicine. 2017;**114**(5):363-366. Available from: https://pubmed.ncbi.nlm.nih.gov/30228634/

[44] Adamson K, Ashcroft R, Langlois S, Lising D. Integrating social work into interprofessional education: A review of one university's curriculum to prepare students for collaborative practice in healthcare. Advances in Social Work. 2020;**20**(2):454-472. DOI: 10.18060/23602

[45] Ogunyemi D, Dupras D. Does an Objective Structured Clinical Examination fit your assessment toolbox? Journal of Graduate Medical Education. 2017;**9**(6):771-772. DOI: 10.4300/JGME-D-17-00655.1

[46] Baharvand P, Nazer MR. The assessment of 360-degree instrument's validity and reliability for evaluation of medical students' performance. Journal of Medical Education Development. 2013;**5**(9):1-6. Available from: http://edujournal.zums.ac.ir/article-1-100-en.html

[47] Cohen DA, Olveczky DD, Tibbles C, Hall MM, Crocker JT. Leading the charge: Effectiveness of a workshop to enhance faculty education of health inequity. The Journal of Continuing Education in the Health Professions. 2023;**43**(1):68-71. DOI: 10.1097/CEH.0000000000000446

[48] Siegel J, Coleman DL, James T. Integrating social determinants of health into graduate medical education: A call for action. Academic Medicine. 2018;**93**(2):159-162. DOI: 10.1097/ACM.0000000000002054

[49] Hasnain M, Darcy-Mahoney A. Let's not reinvent the wheel: Using communities of learning and practice to address SDOH and advance health equity. Annals of Family Medicine. 2023;**21**(Suppl. 2):S95-S99. DOI: 10.1370/afm.2917

[50] Rockey NG, Weiskittel TM, Linder KE, Ridgeway JL, Wieland ML. A mixed methods study to evaluate the impact of a student-run clinic on undergraduate medical education. BMC Medical Education. 2021;**21**:1-9

[51] Moffett SE, Shahidi H, Sule H, Lamba S. Social determinants of health curriculum integrated into a core emergency medicine clerkship. MedEdPORTAL. 2019;**15**:10789

[52] Addy CL, Browne T, Blake EW, Bailey J. Enhancing interprofessional

education: Integrating public health and social work perspectives. American Journal of Public Health. 2015;**105**(Suppl. 1):S106-S108

[53] Drake C, Keeport M, Chapman A, Chakraborti C. Social contexts in medicine: A patient-centered curriculum empowering medical students to provide contextualized care. MedEdPORTAL. 2017;**13**:10541

[54] Gonzalez CM, Fox AD, Marantz PR. The evolution of an elective in health disparities and advocacy: Description of instructional strategies and program evaluation. Academic Medicine. 2015;**90**:1636

[55] Denizard-Thompson N, Palakshappa D, Vallevand A, Kundu D, Brooks A, DiGiacobbe G, et al. Association of a health equity curriculum with medical students' knowledge of social determinants of health and confidence in working with underserved populations. JAMA Network Open. 2021;**4**:e210297

[56] Gimpel N, Kindratt T, Dawson A, Pagels P. Community action research track: Community-based participatory research and service-learning experiences for medical students. Perspectives on Medical Education. 2018;**7**(2):139-143. DOI: 10.1007/s40037-017-0397-2

[57] McNeal MS, Buckner AV. Using mini-grants and service-learning projects to prepare students to serve underserved populations. Journal of Health Care for the Poor and Underserved. 2012;**23**(Suppl. 2):20-26. DOI: 10.1353/hpu.2012.0073

[58] Oriol NE. Celebrating 25 years of transforming care delivery. Health Commune. 2017;**2**:100078. DOI: 10.4172/2472-1654.100078

[59] University of Michigan National Center for Institutional Diversity. Social Determinants of Health Booklet. Ann Arbor, MI: University of Michigan. Available from: https://lsa.umich.edu/content/dam/ncid-assets/ncid-documents/publications/Social%20Determinants%20of%20Health%20Booklet.pdf

[60] Lowery K, Shi L, Weiner JP, Patow C. Money, mission, and medicine: An innovative managed care partnership between the community health centers of Maryland and Johns Hopkins University. The Journal of Ambulatory Care Management. 1999;**22**(4):13-27. DOI: 10.1097/00004479-199910000-00005

[61] Sandella JM, Gimpel JR, Smith LL, Boulet JR. The use of COMLEX-USA and USMLE for residency applicant selection. Journal of Graduate Medical Education. 2016;**8**(3):358-363. DOI: 10.4300/JGME-D-15-00246.1

[62] Adams MC, Denizard-Thompson NM, DiGiacobbe G, Williams BL, Brooks AK. Designing actionable solutions and curriculum for pain disparities education. Pain Medicine. 2022;**23**(2):288-294. DOI: 10.1093/pm/pnab289

[63] Lipshutz JA, Hall JE, Penman-Aguilar A, Skillen E, Naoom S, Irune I. Leveraging social and structural determinants of health at the Centers for Disease Control and Prevention: A systems-level opportunity to improve public health. Journal of Public Health Management and Practice. 2022;**28**(2):E380-E389. DOI: 10.1097/PHH.0000000000001363

[64] Hill C. Using a simulation to increase awareness of the impact of poverty on health care. Journal of Continuing Education in Nursing. 2022;**53**(2):57-58. DOI: 10.3928/00220124-20220104-04

[65] Goetz C, Arora VM, Press VG. Teaching health policy to residents. Journal of General Internal Medicine. 2010;**25**(5):382. DOI: 10.1007/s11606-010-1267-3

[66] Byham JC, Martinez-Gomez V, Kilburn JC Jr, Hilburn AM. When government is not the solution: The role of community organizations in outreach. Journal of Public and Nonprofit Affairs. 2023;**9**(1):4-27. DOI: 10.20899/jpna.9.1.4-27

[67] Kushner J, McConnell KJ. Addressing social determinants of health through Medicaid: Lessons from Oregon. Journal of Health Politics, Policy and Law. 2019;**44**(6):919-935. DOI: 10.1215/03616878-7785823

Chapter 7

Health Literacy Education from Pediatrics to Geriatrics: A Medical Education Perspectives

Valerie A. Ubbes

Abstract

Many premedical and predental students enter undergraduate schools for a liberal education and a preparatory curriculum in medicine or dentistry. These early educational experiences may not address the developmental role of health literacy across the lifespan depending upon which college or school that the preprofessionals took their major. Sometimes health promotion principles may be overlooked as foundational to medical and dental education. Health literacy and health communication are germane topics within all these disciplines and are especially grounded in the education and literacy fields. Health literacy education remains important in the career development of all health professionals from pediatrics to geriatrics. Faculty must interrogate and help preprofessionals to make inferences from literacy and language competencies from which identity and agency emerges across the lifespan. This chapter underscores why national and international literacy data cannot be overlooked when educating professionals about health literacy in medicine and dentistry.

Keywords: health literacy education, developmental perspective, health perspective, literacy perspective, interprofessional perspective, emergent literacy, functional health literacy, interactive health literacy

1. Introduction

Educating for health literacy is a logical advancement in the health literacy field. Faculty teaching in schools of medicine, dentistry, and other health professions are important advocates and decision makers for including health literacy education in higher education curricula [1–3]. For decades, health literacy has been discussed as a theoretical and practical approach for understanding health promotion and disease prevention. Health literacy surveys have been developed to explore the reasons that patients present to hospitals and clinics with widening knowledge gaps and insufficient skills for managing their conditions and diseases. A scoping review of assessment tools for measuring health literacy and digital health literacy in hospital settings found that routine health literacy assessments are still not a part of standard clinical practice [4] even though some medical schools [5] and dental schools [6] report ways to implement a health literacy curriculum with preclinical, clinical, and residency practitioners. Another scoping review investigated the relevancy of health literacy in ensuring effective patient-physician communication [7], coupled with international research showing that health literacy can be explained as a social gradient in childhood, adolescence, and adulthood [8, 9] and as a midstream determinant of health [10]. Medical education is still in need of a concise way to address the multiple sectors, domains, and skills that represent health literacy education. Prioritized health literacy competencies and clear communication practices for health care professionals have been refined in the U.S. [1] with first-time investigations summarized in Europe [11].

One goal of this chapter is to address why health literacy is about literacy-based strategies (i.e., reading, writing, speaking, listening) when accessing valid and reliable information, products, and services about health. This chapter will not address other narratives about information literacy or scientific literacy, which are largely transdisciplinary terms and practices from an academic perspective. The main focus of this chapter is health literacy, because it's a term that crosses multiple sectors of health care, health promotion and disease prevention, and because it's both an interdisciplinary and cross-disciplinary term that explicitly addresses the noun of literacy and the adjective of health. Medical and dental faculty could help their early career students to critically study this lexicon, so they learn to recognize low literacy skills and low health actions among their patients and clients. Practitioners must interact with their clients and patients with valid and reliable health information, products, and services so they will practice health behaviors that have a reciprocal effect on their cognitive and social skills to further enhance their health literacy. An early definition of health literacy ([12], p. 261, 263) suggested that health literacy included "the cognitive and social skills which determine the motivation and ability of individuals to gain access to understand and use information in ways which promote and maintain good health". Researchers continue to investigate ways that cognitive ability may explain the association between health literacy and self-management behaviors [13].

2. Methodology

This chapter uses a narrative review methodology with a focus on three major themes. The first theme will focus on the premise that health literacy education needs to be grounded in a *developmental* perspective. The second theme will focus on the premise that health literacy education needs to be grounded in a *literacy* perspective. And the third theme will focus on the premise that health literacy education needs to be grounded in a *health* perspective. By emphasizing that the second and third themes are an addition and not a replacement to the interdisciplinary term, health literacy, faculty can zoom in on the two concepts of health literacy - first the noun of literacy, then secondly, the adjective of health - to support a fuller understanding for why health literacy initiatives have not been successful in a majority of cases [14]. This chapter augments what faculty are already doing to advance the topic of health literacy in medical and dental schools and encourages faculty to consider an interprofessional perspective on health literacy education.

3. Health literacy education needs a developmental perspective

Medical education needs a developmental framework for determining if individuals have the motivations and skills to demonstrate health literacy from pediatrics to geriatrics. Although a recent scoping review found that citations for health literacy existed for adolescent, young adult, middle adulthood, adult, and aged populations [7], no citations were available for children and only two citations existed for adolescents in that review. Although that same review found that patients and primary care physicians were the foci of a majority of research articles from seven databases published between January 2010 to May 2023, no citations focused on medical education with no specific guidelines for faculty working with early career doctors or dentists. Assuming that current faculty may not have received a medical education in health literacy unless their own research agendas motivated that, a paradigm shift is needed for interdisciplinary study in health literacy. As in the case of health literacy, the fields of health and literacy require "mental flexibility to shift rapidly from one disciplinary perspective to another" and this requires that "the lenses of one discipline are taken off and the lenses of another discipline are put on in their place" ([15], p. 255). Klein argues that program faculty should bear the burden of this sophisticated thinking and practice work:

> *Self-synthesis, the assumption that students can integrate materials and ideas themselves, is inadequate. Synthesis does not occur by osmosis....Students shall not be expected to integrate anything the faculty cannot or will not ([16], p. 54–55, as cited in [17], p. 214).*

Health literacy can be taught from a developmental perspective. A developmental perspective is both psychological and physiological in nature. As the brain grows and matures, the physical frame with all its sophisticated body systems also ages and matures developmentally. The concept of aging employs both a developmental and sociological perspective [18]. The field of developmental psychology investigates the human lifespan while examining physical, cognitive, and social emotional development which has also been adopted by the field of health education. The latter has traditionally employed a lifespan perspective based on the developmental needs and health interests of individuals and groups. Some health educators have advocated for health literacy to be further defined and assessed in quality school health education [19], even though health education instruction has been waning over the years, crippled most recently by the global COVID-19 pandemic which caused ethical dilemmas for all teachers' selfcare and mental health [20]. Beginning in 1995, public schools in the United States addressed the term "health literacy" in the National Health Education Standards document with expanded guidelines for how children and youth could benefit from an age-appropriate, skill-based health education curriculum. An updated *developmental* perspective for health literacy was recently released by the National Consensus for School Health Education [21]. The National Health Education Standards (3rd Edition), in total and in part, may have import to university students exploring careers in all sectors of medicine, dentistry, and health professions because preprofessional students may not have been exposed to the eight curriculum standards and their performance expectations before entering premedical and predental programs in higher education. As such, preprofessional students may not have practiced or learned how to demonstrate functional and interactive health literacy across the pre-kindergarten to grade 12 curriculum. This means that there could be a real lag in demonstrating and even comprehending what health literacy is all about from a developmental perspective.

Health literacy education should include study on the role of identity in literacy development. Identity is "actively formed through the practice of clarifying goals, assessing skills, and developing plans to reach goals. Such practices operate through building professional and personal networks, as well as articulating the purpose of one's work to a broader audience" [22]. Feeling that one's identity and goals fit within a particular environment fosters a sense of authenticity [23]. Therefore, constructing a coherent self as a doctor or dentist requires an understanding of literacy research that is set into a broader context of practice settings, including one's participation in a medical or dental curriculum that deepens the personal, cognitive, and social development of health literacy skills.

Cultural intersections are also important to study and understand in health literacy education. Human identities are often characterized by gender, class, ethnicity, and age [18] with multiple identities intersecting to make each person unique. These identities emerge when individuals communicate through language and multimodal literacies [24]. For example, national [25] and international studies [26] show that girls have more positive attitudes toward reading than boys with these trends continuing into adulthood. Medical and dental curricula should also address the intersection between literacy, class, and ethnicities. Lower income populations often lack the financial supports and literacy-rich environments necessary for encouraging reading and dual language programs. Differences exist in reading skills among ethnic populations such as Caucasians and Asians who have more advanced reading skills than other minorities [27]. Literacy practices extend beyond reading. Writing and speaking have been added to the health literacy skillset to round out the developmental abilities of students for functional health literacy and interactive health literacy ([21], p. 11–12).

Medical and dental students require a developmental perspective as they advance through their health literacy education. Students can be encouraged to read peer-review journal articles outside of medicine and dentistry to study national and international literacy trends for themselves. In peer-led, smaller learning communities, students should explore literacy, education, and public health research to more fully understand gendered, minoritized, economic, and environmental perspectives that often affect people's lived experiences with literacy, language, and health literacy – or their lack thereof. Faculty can then facilitate larger group discussions to uncover any biases and false stereotypes that their medical and dental students may have assumed when attending to patients and clients in a health care clinic during their training. By opening windows of time in the health literacy curriculum for student storytelling and discussion, the professionals themselves construct meaning through the language they use to explain (or write about) any misconceptions they may have about the language and literacy practices of others. These health literacy discussions enable the professional identities of the doctor(s) and dentist(s) to develop more fully into an intentional plan for empowerment, so their autonomy and self-determination emerge. Faculty can be encouraged to know that "For underrepresented students, the presence of other group members can relieve stereotypic expectations, foster better engagement and performance. Even one other person with a shared identity can make a difference...Knowing oneself and one's field requires knowing others immersed in different fields or contexts because identifying both similarities and differences in others' experiences allows students to see their own values and contexts more clearly. In this framework, professional identity is constructed through repeated practices of coming together with others..." ([22], p. 5).

The medical curriculum at the University of South Carolina School of Medicine Greenville [5] provides an example for highlighting the importance of professional identity formation in their first semester block. The first semester block focuses on the intrapersonal and interpersonal levels of the ecological model with the topics of health literacy, professional identity formation, systems thinking, communication, evidence-based practice, and other topics. The second semester block focuses on the organizational level of the ecological model with such topics as access to care, teaming and communication, and care settings and coordination. And the third semester block focuses on the public and community levels of the ecological model with cultural competence, bias in healthcare, and healthcare leadership and advocacy as three of the six topics included.

3.1 Health literacy education needs a literacy perspective

This section will focus on a *literacy perspective* in the context of health literacy education. Medical and dental students are dependent upon the pedagogies and practices of faculty to uncover and explore more deeply the *literacy* needs of people as the *sine qua non* of health literacy. Literacy is the common throughline across all the professional practice settings where health literacy is important. As such, literacy practices need to be elucidated for their contributions to health literacy. This means that faculty in medical and dental schools need support in seeing that the disciplinary work they do every day is a literacy practice. All professionals use language and literacy to draw meaning from the texts, subtexts, and contexts of their medical, dental, and health professions practice.

From where do the inspirations to become medical and dental professionals come? How do literacy scores and access to literacy-rich environments help to play a role? According to the 2022 National Assessment of Educational Progress (NAEP), two-thirds of fourth graders in the United States are reading at a basic or below level [28]. NAEP data also show that U.S. teens grow up with gendered differences in reading and writing achievement [29]. This may be important to discuss and problem solve when youth age into adulthood without the ability "to demonstrate health literacy by accessing valid and reliable health information, products, or services" as sequenced by grade-level performance expectations in the National Health Education Standards [21, 30]. Recent improvements in outlining functional and interactive health literacy skills may help administrators, educators, and health professionals to promote the preK-12 developmental skillset needed to advance health literacy in the United States.

International literacy and global reading concerns are worth addressing in the medical and dental curriculum as well. Lower overall literacy scores in the U.S. means that health literacy will also be lower. In 2021, the Progress in International Reading Literacy Study (PIRLS) [31] determined that 10 countries had end-of-fourth grade literacy assessments higher than the United States. These countries included (in order) Singapore, Ireland, Hong Kong, Russian Federation, Northern Ireland, England, Croatia, Lithuania, Finland, and Poland. The United States was next followed by Chinese Taipei (Taiwan), Sweden, Australia, Bulgaria, and Czech Republic. Of the top 10 countries, Ireland, Northern Ireland, Croatia, Lithuania, and the United States delayed their fourth grade reading assessments until the beginning of fifth grade.

A concept like literacy is a mental representation that is understood (or not) from one's own background knowledge. If one lacks background knowledge about illiteracy and has had few practical connections with low literacy patients, then it is unlikely that the conception of health literacy for an early professional will be addressed or appreciated in an adequate way. Similarly, if the early career student has been an excellent consumer of both digital media and print media because of being surrounded by peers who were highly literate and articulate in prior schooling, then the preprofessional may need even more modules to learn the subtleties of patient culture and linguistic backgrounds. The National Standards for Culturally and Linguistically Appropriate Services in Health Care (CLAS) [32] provide an excellent backdrop to health literacy education, because the standards were written to reduce racial and ethnic health disparities in clinical care and public health [33]. Faculty can guide their preprofessional students to be responsive to diverse cultural beliefs and practices, preferred languages, health literacy, and other communication needs of their patients [32].

Young people who grow up to be adult readers have a life-long disadvantage because they have a smaller vocabulary in their first language and even less proficiency in their second or third language. When these same children and youth become adults, a health and medical lexicon remains missing in their language development which also supports their literacy development. For example, if children or youth have had limited reading or speaking opportunities, they may also lack concepts for building a background knowledge in health and medicine. Zwaan and Brown [34] argue that language and vocabulary proficiencies affect the number and kind of inferences that readers generate. Individuals who have lacked literacy-rich environments and/or literature centered approaches to health and medicine in their upbringing will not be able to retrieve information from either prior texts or background knowledge to understand what is being discussed. Shifting the focus to how patients understand something by encouraging them to put information into their own words will assist clinicians in making healthcare decisions with their patients. This mutuality in health communications and health literacy can result in a stronger identity formation and agency for patients.

Students learning about health literacy in medical and dental schools could study and participate in two national pediatric programs that focus on book distributions to families: Reach Out and Read and Imagination Library. The Reach Out and Read program with over 6000 clinical sites has decades of support in establishing the value of early literacy practices among children and their parents [35]. The Reach Out and Read program recognizes emergent literacy [35]. Emergent literacy is a strong predictor of reading abilities and problems as a child ages [36]. Emergent literacy is foundational to functional health literacy and interactive health literacy in children with each type of health literacy supporting identity development and agency, respectively [24]. Emergent literacy includes a broad range of pre-literacy skills, knowledge, and attitudes [37] and spoken language, print knowledge, and phonological processing abilities [38]. Some pediatricians have proposed that literacy become the fifth recognized domain of child development because reading and writing requires practice and rehearsal of multiple neural networks through direct instruction, unlike oral language which is already an emergent language hardwired in the brain as an innate ability [35]. The American Academy of Pediatrics [39] recently established a policy statement making literacy promotion and reading aloud essential components of primary care pediatric practice and the recognition of literacy as a social driver of health.

Reach Out and Read claims that only 1 in 3 children under age two are read to every day – and only 1 in 4 kids from households with low incomes are read to every day. As a result, families may not read together as a daily routine, which means that children will miss out on important opportunities to build their essential language and listening skills through conversations and socioemotional bonding around books. By the year 2030, Reach Out and Read has plans to serve 10 million kids – which represents one-half of all children under age 5 in the United States. Today, Reach Out and Read serves 4.6 million children who receive a free developmentally appropriate book each time they meet with their pediatrician for a well-child checkup between the ages of 6 months and 5 years.

Another important book distribution program includes Imagination Library which was established by the singer, Dolly Parton, who mails children one free picture book each month until their fifth birthday for a total of 60 books. Any child in a participating U.S. state is eligible to receive books for a home library between birth and age five [40, 41]. Pediatric programs like Reach Out and Read and Imagination Library continue to be successful in providing books for establishing home libraries for children. Medical researchers in a midwestern U.S. city found that preschoolers who were given books from both the Reach Out and Read program and the Imagination Library program were significantly better at speech and language development, preliteracy skills, and kindergarten readiness scores when compared to children receiving books from only one program or no programs [42]. Evidence-based programs like Reach Out and Read provide parents and caregivers with encouragement to read to their children everyday using prosocial skills and interactive language-rich conversations about books. When grandparents and parents read aloud to children at home, an intergenerational connection is fostered between the young and old while developing emergent literacy and language skills.

Boosts to oral health literacy have been proposed as viable pediatric programs in dental clinics [43] and school-based health clinics [44] for elementary students. Moving toward literature-based dentistry can be one way to boost health literacy and oral health literacy of children through interprofessional partnerships between dentists, doctors, and librarians [43]. Such interprofessional partnerships advance the expectation that infants should have a dental home by age 1 enhanced by a stronger pediatric referral process between dentists and pediatricians and the need to educate parents and their children about daily oral hygiene practices and 6 month dental checkups for disease prevention. An eBook for Oral Health Literacy© curriculum [45] and its accompanying workbook, website, and social media platforms offer evidence-based oral hygiene stories for school-age children [44], their parents [46], and teachers [47].

Other successful literacy programs exist across the developmental lifespan. Adult literacy is critical for those in low income populations or in minoritized populations who may have multilinguistic needs. There are good models of community health organizations and federally qualified health centers teaming with Adult Basic Education (ABE) programs in Florida, New York City, Chicago, and Boston [48]. Because research has linked low literacy and limited English with poorer health, adult basic education programs have offered health literacy programs along with preventive health screenings for adult learners. This integration of health literacy programs with English Language Learners is important because 22 percent or 67 million people speak a language other than English at home, and 8 percent or 25.6 million Americans have limited English proficiency (LEP) [49]. Adult populations with lower rates of health literacy are also likely to have limited access to the Internet so some adult basic education programs are also forming partnerships to help adults learn digital health literacy skills [50].

Low health literacy is a threat to the health and wellbeing of adults and children [51]. Health literacy can be compromised when functional health is lacking from birth or deteriorating from the adult aging process. Health professionals in both the medical and dental sectors need to address the cognitive changes that accompany sensiomotor deficits in vision [52], hearing loss [53], and poor oral health [54] in older adults over the age of 65 years. These cognitive changes play a significant role in memory and literacy abilities, including adults' ability to manage their health. On the other end of the aging spectrum, research shows that approximately 1 out of every 6 children has been diagnosed with one or more developmental disabilities in the U.S. between 2009 and 2017 prior to the COVID-19 pandemic [55]. Developmental disabilities of children are lifelong conditions that could include impairments or delays in their physical health, learning ability, language ability, or behaviors. Specific developmental disabilities include attention-deficit hyperactivity disorder; autism spectrum disorder; blindness; cerebral palsy; moderate to profound hearing loss; learning disability; intellectual disability; seizures; stuttering or stammering; and other developmental delays.

Part of the reason that so many adults are not able to demonstrate adequate reading skills can be inferred from the leading health indicators provided by *Healthy People 2030* [28]. In 2017, only 36.6 percent of 4th grade students attending public and private schools in the U.S. had reading skills at or above the proficient achievement level for their grade. However, in 2022, a lower 33.3 percent of 4th grade students attending public and private schools in the U.S. had reading skills at or above the proficient achievement level for their grade. Unfortunately, these data indicate that a majority of fourth graders are not reading at grade level, and the results have gotten worse during the 5 year interval (which included the insult of the coronavirus pandemic). When children and youth have learned to read, they have the potential to grow up to be successful readers as adults. If there are higher rates of adults who are learning to read for the first time (as adults) this means that they did not learn to read during their elementary and secondary school years - and that remains a practical problem for health literacy.

One thought experiment for developing health literacy is borrowed from work by Ne'eman and Shaul [56], who found a very strong association between cognitive measures and literacy measures among kindergarten children. Different cognitive skills like naming, working memory, executive functioning, and information processing speed explained 51 percent of the variance in emergent literacy tests. Because cognitive abilities and emergent literacy skills appear to covary, a future longitudinal study is necessary to examine this cognition-literacy connection across a wide range of populations with different backgrounds and abilities. As we turn to a health perspective in the next section, what might be the role of health behaviors in boosting cognitive ability? Researchers ([56], p. 17) state: "...it may be necessary to more thoroughly develop curriculum programs that enhance cognitive abilities, by improving the information processing rate, executive abilities, and inhibition as well as memory abilities from an early age". Can health behaviors play a role in enhancing these cognitive abilities toward health literacy?

3.2 Health literacy education needs a health perspective

Although the last section addressed the disabilities and conditions that serve as barriers to literacy when working with children and adults in clinical care, this section will now focus on a *health perspective* in the context of health literacy education. Research serves as a useful bridge in understanding that a decrease in cognitive functioning is related to limited health literacy [57]. When doctors and dentists understand that pediatric and geriatric cognitive functioning can be associated with a person's functional health and functional health literacy, more research can be established to look at the effects of certain health behaviors on cognitive health and literacy. As the 10 year cognitive functioning study [57] has suggested: "Older adults with poorer cognitive functioning and stronger cognitive decline are at risk for having low health literacy, which can affect their abilities to promote health and self-manage disease. Low health literacy and declining cognitive functioning might be a barrier for person-centered care, even in relatively young older adults". Therefore, there would be benefits in faculty promoting a few health-enhancing behaviors like sleep, nutrition, and physical activity for building cognitive vitality and literacy in tandem. Examples could include: 1) the positive effects of sleep on cognitive health and literacy [58], the positive effects of nutrition on cognitive health and literacy [59]; and 3) the positive effects of physical activity on cognitive health and literacy [60, 61].

The International Union for Health Promotion and Education [62] has a practical vision for a health literate world because health literacy is "viewed as an important outcome of health promotion interventions" (p. 14). Their IUHPE Position Statement on Health Literacy [63] addresses health literacy as a social determinant of health with a need to integrate health literacy into clinical practice and public health interventions across the lifespan. The IUHPE is a global professional non-governmental organization dedicated to health promotion around the world for more than 70 years. The IUHPE [64] states that "Health education is most likely to improve health literacy when the messaging and delivery are tailored to the specific needs of individuals and populations across their life course", and when the interventions are "linked to critical life stages (e.g., adolescence, parenthood, aging and retirement) and events (e.g., diagnosis of chronic disease)" (p. 15). When health literacy is seen as an intervention to support greater personal autonomy, autonomy in this context refers to the individual's agency to change, adapt, communicate, make decisions and do goal-directed behaviors for their health.

3.3 Health literacy education needs an interprofessional perspective

This section promotes an interprofessional perspective that depends upon faculty members who use medicine and dentistry as the vehicles to advance health literacy education as a developmental skillset for accessing valid and reliable health information, products, and services across the lifespan. An interprofessional perspective refers to interactions, collaborations, and activities that involve individuals from different professions or disciplines working together with a common goal. In healthcare, this involves health workers from different professional backgrounds working together with patients, families, communities to deliver health care and promote health literacy.

An important step for health literacy education in medicine and dentistry would be the two fields working side by side to collaborate on the improvement of global health equity [65]. Even though medicine and dentistry have their own schools for preparing the next generation of doctors and dentists, there are ample reasons for new interprofessional curricula to consider oral health an integral part of general health at the undergraduate, graduate, and postgraduate levels of education [65]. By overlapping the medical and dental curricula worldwide, the interdisciplinary approaches will afford dentists the ability to recognize early detection of non-communicable and infectious diseases and help doctors to promote the 2021 WHO recommendation that poor oral health is a major contributor to respiratory diseases, sleep-related breathing disorders, and cognitive decline [66]. Basic facts like the mouth being an integral part of the digestive and respiratory tract, and infants needing a dental home by age one are important principles for advancing integrative patient care.

Medical and dental faculty could use health literacy educational approaches [67] and establish a constructivist learning environment which helps health professionals to generate critical and creative thinking [68] and develop oral language skills for enhancing their health communication competencies [69]. As explained by Jonassen ([70] p. 36), "Constructivist environments facilitate learning through collaboration, context, and construction of knowledge. Through assimilation and accommodation, individuals use many elements of the learning context and relate those elements to their own experiences, thus creating new knowledge". This philosophy would be an excellent way to grow the health literacy curriculum in medical and dental schools while using the lived experiences of the medical and dental students. All health professionals could help to advocate for more exposure to health literacy standards in preK-12 schools and in preprofessional curricula in universities before medical and dental students get into their professional training. Advocacy from the current medical and dental students can help to strengthen the health literacy agenda across the developmental lifespan and help them to develop a health literacy capstone in medical and dental schools. A promising health literacy capstone could address digital health literacy and the role of technology in health care. For example, a recent scoping review found that healthcare professionals still need more health literacy continuing education courses and tools for supporting and communicating with older patients who have limited health literacy skills [71]. Hence, students could explore how age is an essential risk factor for lower health literacy and determine how their use of technology might enhance or hinder older people as they age.

Service learning would be a vital way to implement a health literacy module into the curriculum for early career students in medical and dental school [72] suggests that practitioners, who collaborate with literacy coalitions to coteach health literacy courses in adult education programs, would be a valuable service learning project with a win-win outcome. This could also afford medical and dental schools the opportunity to partner with family, health, and social service agencies for more authentic experiences in health literacy theory and practice.

Faculty in medical and dental schools need to model the role of health literacy in their own work. Health literacy includes talking and writing about health and literacy topics through forums, podcasts, and professional organizations. Faculty should encourage their students to go to conferences to speak about their experiences with health literacy and to submit health literacy manuscripts to professional journals. At minimum, students should be reading from the vast health literacy research and summarizing it in class in small groups. When students are asked to present professional case studies to their peers and colleagues, they practice health literacy skills along with critical and creative thinking skills. Developmental thinking processes can be scaffolded when faculty teach about health literacy using Bloom's Taxonomy [73] as an explicit way to probe lower to higher levels of cognition. This thinking practice may give students insights into why they are able to advance through medical or dental school while others may be lacking in cognitive skills and subsequently challenged by functional and interactive health literacy skills.

Faculty use of an inquiry-based pedagogy to foster self-authorship among medical and dental students could also prove promising. The Stages of Cognitive Development model [74] outlines learners who move through absolute, transitional, independent, and contextual stages of identity and autonomy. Faculty could investigate how their early career students vary along the Stages of Cognitive Development model toward self-authorship. In this context, self-authorship may have the potential to serve as a proxy for career readiness in health literacy competencies. To support students in their developing cognitive abilities in medical and dental education, faculty could also use inquiry-based strategies like written questions, cues, prompts, and comparisons between functional health literacy, interactive health literacy, and critical health literacy to generate research projects.

Finally, writing is an integral skill that serves a metacognitive purpose in health literacy education. According to Hacker et al. ([75], p. 170), "Writing can be a solitary cognitive act of producing meaning for oneself, and writing can be a social act of producing meaning through negotiation with others". In order to provoke students to think about thinking in a metacognitive way, faculty can use think-aloud protocols and directed retrospection with "investigative writing at the moment of production" to get to the "production of meaning that results from a person's goal-directed monitoring and control of their cognitive and affective states". Faculty could generate writing tasks to negotiate the topic and practice of health literacy within solo and small groups of early and late career students using one or two of the following examples:

- Write a developmental argument for building stronger cognitive memory skills for children and adults;
- Write scenarios or a case study for describing how culturally and linguistically appropriate care and services will be put into your medical or dental practice;
- Write scripts for promoting reading in doctor and dental offices for pediatric patients and geriatric patients;
- Write about the value of having all members of your clinical team to promote health literacy in daily health care practices; or
- Write about one of the standards or policy documents described in this chapter that can be implemented and sustained in the health literacy education curriculum in medical and dental schools.

4. Conclusion

Health literacy education remains important in the career development of all health professionals from pediatrics to geriatrics. To advance health literacy education, a literacy perspective, a health perspective, and an interprofessional perspective are needed as foundational building blocks to professional knowledge. Faculty need to teach a developmental perspective when supporting their early and late career students to develop their own literacy and language competencies from which professional identity and agency emerges. Understanding the literacy and health research across the developmental lifespan brings health literacy into reality when interacting with patients across the lifespan.

Conflict of interest

The author declares no conflict of interest.

Author details

Valerie A. Ubbes
Miami University, Oxford, OH, USA

*Address all correspondence to: ubbesva@miamioh.edu

References

[1] Coleman C, Hudson S, Pederson B. Prioritized health literacy and clear communication practices for health care professionals. HLRP: Health Literacy Research and Practice. 2017;**1**(3):e91-e99. DOI: 10.3928/24748307-20170503-01

[2] Felter NJ, Ubbes VA. A descriptive study of health literacy and social determinants of health as curricula topics in medical school education. Health Behavior Research. 2023;**6**(1):1. DOI: 10.4148/2572-1836.1160

[3] Ubbes VA, Njoku B. A curriculum, instruction, and assessment (CIA) framework for health literacy education (HLE) in medical and health professions schools. World Journal of Social Science Research. 2022;**9**(1):1-41. DOI: 10.22158/wjssr.v9n1p15

[4] Dijkman EM, Brake WWM, Drossaert CHC, Doggen CJM. Assessment tools for measuring. Health literacy and digital health literacy in a hospital setting: A scoping review. Healthcare. 2024;**12**(1):11. DOI: 10.3390/healthcare12010011

[5] Albertson F, Kennedy AB, Taylor SS, Natafgi N. Evaluating medical learners' experiences with health literacy at a southeastern medical school. BMC Medical Education. 2025;**25**(1):23. DOI: 10.1186/s12909-024-06362-6

[6] Maybury C, Williams MA, Challenger K, Fassas E, Galvan S, Gelmann D, et al. How health literacy is taught and evaluated in dentistry, medicine, nursing, law, pharmacy, public health, and social work: A narrative review. Journal of Communication in Healthcare. 2024;**17**(1):51-67. DOI: 10.1080/17538068.2023.2258315

[7] Vamos SD, Vine ME, Gordon ID, Alaimo DF. The role of health literacy in patient-physician communication: A scoping review. Health Behavior and Policy Review. 2024;**11**(4):1624-1654. DOI: 10.14485/HBPR.11.4.2

[8] Bröder J, Okan O, Bauer U, Schlupp S, Pinheiro P. Advancing perspectives on health literacy in childhood and youth. Health Promotion International. 2020;**35**(3):575-585. DOI: 10.1093/heapro/daz041

[9] Sørensen K, Van den Broucke S, Fullam J, Doyle G, Pelikan J, Slonska Z, et al. Health literacy and public health: A systematic review and integration of definitions and models. BMC Public Health. 2012;**12**:1-3. DOI: 10.1186/1471-2458-12-80

[10] Nutbeam D, Lloyd JE. Understanding and responding to health literacy as a social determinant of health. Annual Review of Public Health. 2021;**42**(1):159-173. DOI: 10.1146/annurev-publhealth-090419-102529

[11] Karuranga S, Sørensen K, Coleman C, Mahmud AJ. Health literacy competencies for European health care personnel. HLRP: Health Literacy Research and Practice. 2017;**1**(4):e247-e256. DOI: 10.3928/24748307-20171005-01

[12] Nutbeam D. Health literacy as a public health goal: A challenge for contemporary health education and communication strategies into the 21st century. Health Promotion International. 2000;**15**(3):259-267. DOI: 10.1093/heapro/15.3.259

[13] O'Conor R, Wolf MS, Smith SG, Martynenko M, Vicencio DP, Sano M,

et al. Health literacy, cognitive function, proper use, and adherence to inhaled asthma controller medications among older adults with asthma. Chest. 2015;**147**(5):1307-1315. DOI: 10.1378/chest.14-0914

[14] Hudson S, Rikard RV, Staiculescu I, et al. Improving health and the bottom line: The case for health literacy. In: National Academies of Sciences, Engineering, and Medicine; Health and Medicine Division; Board on Population Health and Public Health Practice; Roundtable on Health Literacy. Building the Case for Health Literacy: Proceedings of a Workshop. Washington (DC): National Academies Press (US); 2018. Appendix C. Available from: https://www.ncbi.nlm.nih.gov/books/NBK518850/

[15] Newell WH. 13 decision making in interdisciplinary studies. In: Morcol G, editor. Handbook of Decision Making. New York: Marcel Dekker; 2007. pp. 245-265

[16] Gaff JG. Avoiding the potholes: Strategies for reforming general education. Educational Record. 1980;**61**(4):50-59

[17] Klein JT. Crossing Boundaries: Knowledge, Disciplinarities, and Interdisciplinarities. Charlottesville, VA: University of Virginia Press; 1996

[18] Hosokawa F. Ageing as a developmental perspective. Journal of Sociology and Social Work. 2016;**4**(2):28-37. DOI: 10.15640/jssw.v4n2a4

[19] Videto DM, Dake JA. Promoting health literacy through defining and measuring quality school health education. Health Promotion Practice. 2019;**20**(6):824-833. DOI: 10.1177/1524839919870194

[20] Gurr SK, Geron T, Forster DJ, Levinson M. Philosophical reflections on teachers' ethical dilemmas in a global pandemic. Studies in Philosophy and Education. 2024;**44**:187-207. DOI: 10.1007/s11217-024-09937-4

[21] National Consensus for School Health Education. National Health Education Standards: Model Guidance for Curriculum and Instruction. 3rd ed. 2022. Available from: www.schoolhealtheducation.org

[22] Diekman AB, Ward RM, Yezierski EJ, Bretz SL. Developing identity via intentional interdisciplinary engagement: Exploring new mentoring models for STEM graduate students' professional development. Mentoring & Tutoring: Partnership in Learning. 2025:1-21. DOI: 10.1080/13611267.2024.2441125

[23] Schmader T, Sedikides C. State authenticity as fit to environment: The implications of social identity for fit, authenticity, and self-segregation. Personality and Social Psychology Review. 2018;**22**(3):228-259. DOI: 10.1177/1088868317734080

[24] Ubbes VA. Emergent Literacy Is Foundational to Health Literacy in Children: Interdisciplinary Relationships to Boost Child Health. London, UK: IntechOpen; 2024. pp. 1-9. DOI: 10.5772/intechopen.113003. ISBN 978-1-83769-247-7

[25] Ubbes VA, Dillhoff R, Maldonado W. Reading and writing attitudes of children: Conceptual implications for health education and health literacy. Journal of Health Education Teaching. 2018;**9**(1):49-67

[26] Scholes L. Differences in attitudes towards reading and other school-related activities among boys and girls. Journal of Research in Reading. 2019;**42**(3-4):485-503. DOI: 10.1111/1467-9817.12279

[27] Carnoy M, García E. Five Key Trends in US Student Performance: Progress by Blacks and Hispanics, the Takeoff of Asians, the Stall of Non-English Speakers, the Persistence of Socioeconomic Gaps, and the Damaging Effect of Highly Segregated Schools. Washington, DC: Economic Policy Institute; 2017

[28] Office of Disease Prevention and Health Promotion. Healthy People 2030. U.S. Department of Health and Human Services; n.d. Available from: https://odphp.health.gov/healthypeople/objectives-and-data/leading-health-indicators

[29] Reilly D, Neumann DL, Andrews G. Gender differences in reading and writing achievement: Evidence from the National Assessment of educational Progress (NAEP). American Psychologist. 2019;**74**(4):445. DOI: 10.1037/amp0000356

[30] Birch DA, McNeill EB, Tappe M, Ubbes VA. National health education standards: Model guidance for curriculum and instruction (third edition). Journal of School Health. 2025;**95**(1):105-112. DOI: 10.1111/josh.13515

[31] Mullis IVS, von Davier M, Foy P, Fishbein B, Reynolds KA, Wry E, et al. International Results in Reading. Chestnut Hill, MA: Boston College, TIMSS & PIRLS International Study Center; 2021. DOI: 10.6017/lse.tpisc.tr2103.kb5342

[32] Williams MV, Martin LT, Davis LM, May LW, Kim A. Evaluation of the National CLAS Standards. Washington, DC: US Department of Health and Human Services Office of Minority Health; 2018. pp. 1-5. Available from: https://mhmrcv.org/wp-content/uploads/2022/11/Evaluation_of_the_Natn_CLAS_Standards_Toolkit_PR3599_final.508Compliant.pdf

[33] Barksdale CL, Rodick WH, Hopson R, Kenyon J, Green K, Jacobs CG. Literature review of the national CLAS standards: Policy and practical implications in reducing health disparities. Journal of Racial and Ethnic Health Disparities. 2017:632-647. DOI: 10.1007/s40615-016-0267-3

[34] Zwaan RA, Brown CM. The influence of language proficiency and comprehension skill on situation-model construction. Discourse Processes. 1996;**21**(3):289-327. DOI: 10.1080/01638539609544960

[35] Klass P, Hutton JS, DeWitt TG. Literacy as a distinct developmental domain in children. JAMA Pediatrics. 2020;**174**(5):407-408. DOI: 10.1001/jamapediatrics.2020.0059

[36] Esmaeeli Z, Kyle FE, Lundetræ K. Contribution of family risk, emergent literacy and environmental protective factors in children's reading difficulties at the end of second grade. Reading and Writing. 2019;**32**(9):2375-2399. DOI: 10.1007/s11145-019-09948-5

[37] Whitehurst GJ, Lonigan CJ. Emergent literacy: Development from prereaders to readers. Handbook of Early Literacy Research. 2001;**1**:11-29

[38] Teale WH, Whittingham CE, Hoffman EB. Early literacy research, 2006-2015: A decade of measured progress. Journal of Early Childhood Literacy. 2020;**20**(2):169-222. DOI: 10.1177/1468798418754939

[39] Klass P, Miller-Fitzwater A, High PC. Literacy promotion: An essential component of primary care

pediatric practice: Policy statement. Pediatrics. 2024;**154**(6):e2024069090

[40] Skibbe LE, Foster TD. Participation in the imagination library book distribution program and its relations to children's language and literacy outcomes in kindergarten. Reading Psychology. 2019;**40**(4):350-370. DOI: 10.1080/02702711.2019.1614124

[41] Stone JK. Reading power with and through Dolly Parton's imagination library: A critical content analysis [dissertation]. Chapel Hill: University of North Carolina; 2024

[42] Szumlas GA, Petronio P, Mitchell MJ, Johnson AJ, Henry TR, DeWitt TG. A combined reach out and read and imagination library program on kindergarten readiness. Pediatrics. 2021;**147**(6):1-9. DOI: 10.1542/peds.2020-027581

[43] Ubbes VA, Miner M, Karthikeyan M. Moving toward literature-based dentistry to boost oral health literacy of children: Interprofessional partnerships between dentists, doctors, and librarians. In: Naomi Lesley N, Hardstaff SL, editors. Health Care in Children's. Media, Jackson, MS: University Press of Mississippi; 2025

[44] Ubbes VA, Miranda MA, McConnell M. Oral health knowledge, reading comprehension, and behavior change after implementing the eBook for Oral health literacy© curriculum with 3rd graders during COVID-19: Implications for school health education. International Electronic Journal of Elementary Education. 2025;**17**(4)

[45] Ubbes VA, Witter AM, Kraska CM, Justus EE. Evaluation of an eBook for oral health literacy© to promote child health: Readability, suitability, understandability, actionability, and gist-based message design. Children and Teenager. 2020;**3**(1):1-27. DOI: 10.22158/ct.v3n1p54

[46] Ubbes VA, Witter A. Parental influences on children's oral health behaviors, reading behaviors, and reading attitudes associated with the sharing of a digital story from the eBook for oral health literacy© curriculum. Children and Teenagers. 2021;**4**(3):26-55. DOI: 10.22158/ct.v4n3p26

[47] Ubbes V, Whitesel S. Use of an eBook for oral health literacy© curriculum to elicit functional health knowledge, decision making, and goal setting among school-aged children. International Electronic Journal of Elementary Education. 2022;**15**(2):145-159. DOI: 10.26822/iejee.2023.286

[48] Hohn MD, Lawrence W, McKinney J, Rosen DJ, Santos MG, Sheppard R, et al. Adult basic education: Community health partnerships and health disparities. HLRP: Health Literacy Research and Practice. 2019;**3**(3):S1-S7. DOI: 10.3928/24748307-20181125-01

[49] Flores G. Language barriers and hospitalized children: Are we overlooking the most important risk factor for adverse events? JAMA Pediatrics. 2020;**174**(12):e203238. DOI: 10.1001/jamapediatrics.2020.3238

[50] Harris K, Jacobs G, Reeder J. Health systems and adult basic education: A critical partnership in supporting digital health literacy. HLRP: Health Literacy Research and Practice. 2019;**3**(3):S33-S36. DOI: 10.3928/24748307-20190325-02

[51] Koenig VE. Health literacy: Pure and simple. Annals of Physiotherapy & Occupational Therapy. 2018;**1**(2):1-3

[52] Lee CS, Gibbons LE, Lee AY, Yanagihara RT, Blazes MS, Lee ML, et al. Association between cataract extraction

and development of dementia. JAMA Internal Medicine. 2022;**182**(2):134-141. DOI: 10.1001/jamainternmed.2021.6990

[53] Yévenes-Briones H, Caballero FF, Struijk EA, Rey-Martinez J, Montes-Jovellar L, Graciani A, et al. Association between hearing loss and impaired physical function, frailty, and disability in older adults: A cross-sectional study. JAMA Otolaryngology–Head & Neck Surgery. 2021;**147**(11):951-958. DOI: 10.1001/jamaoto.2021.2399

[54] Jockusch J, Riese F, Theill N, Sobotta BA, Nitschke I. Aspects of oral health and dementia among Swiss nursing home residents. Zeitschrift für Gerontologie und Geriatrie. 2021;**54**(5):500-506. DOI: 10.1007/s00391-020-01739-w

[55] Zablotsky B, Black LI, Maenner MJ, Schieve LA, Danielson ML, Bitsko RH, et al. Prevalence and trends of developmental disabilities among children in the United States: 2009-2017. Pediatrics. 2019;**144**(4):e20190811. DOI: 10.1542/peds.2019-0811

[56] Ne'eman A, Shaul S. The association between emergent literacy and cognitive abilities in kindergarten children. Child & Youth Care Forum. 2023;**52**(2):467-488. DOI: 10.1007/s10566-022-09697-7

[57] Geboers B, Uiters E, Reijneveld SA, Jansen CJ, Almansa J, Nooyens AC, et al. Health literacy among older adults is associated with their 10-years' cognitive functioning and decline-the Doetinchem Cohort Study. BMC Geriatrics. 2018;**18**:1-7

[58] Åslund L, Arnberg F, Kanstrup M, Lekander M. Cognitive and behavioral interventions to improve sleep in school-age children and adolescents: A systematic review and meta-analysis. Journal of Clinical Sleep Medicine. 2018;**14**(11):1937-1947. DOI: 10.5664/csm.7498

[59] Laurent JS, Watts R, Adise S, Allgaier N, Chaarani B, Garavan H, et al. Associations among body mass index, cortical thickness, and executive function in children. JAMA Pediatrics. 2020;**174**(2):170-177. DOI: 10.1001/jamapediatrics.2019.4708

[60] Lebrun-Harris LA, Ghandour RM, Kogan MD, Warren MD. Five-year trends in US children's health and well-being, 2016-2020. JAMA Pediatrics. 2022;**176**(7):1-11. DOI: 10.1001/jamapediatrics.2022.0056

[61] Buja A, Rabensteiner A, Sperotto M, Grotto G, Bertoncello C, Cocchio S, et al. Health literacy and physical activity: A systematic review. Journal of Physical Activity and Health. 2020;**17**(12):1259-1274. DOI: 10.1123/jpah.2020-0161

[62] International Union of Health Promotion and Education (IUHPE). 2018. Available from: https://iuhpe.org

[63] Bröder J, Chang P, Kickbusch I, Levin-Zamir D, McElhinney E, Nutbeam D, et al. IUHPE position statement on health literacy: A practical vision for a health literate world. In: IUPE Global Working Group on Health Literacy. Paris: IUHPE; 2018

[64] Levin-Zamir D, Nutbeam D, Sorensen K, Rowlands G, Van den Broucke S, Pelikan J, et al. Brief report on the International Union for Health Promotion and Education (IUHPE) position statement on health literacy: A practical vision for a health literate world. Public Health Panorama. 2019;**5**(2-3):206-209

[65] Lobbezoo F, Aarab G. Medicine and dentistry working side by side to improve global health equity. Journal of Dental

Research. 2022;**101**(10):1133-1134. DOI: 10.1177/00220345221088237

[66] Seitz MW, Listl S, Bartols A, Schubert I, Blaschke K, Haux C, et al. Current knowledge on correlations between highly prevalent dental conditions and chronic diseases: An umbrella review. Preventing Chronic Disease. 2019;**2019**(16):180641. DOI: 10.5888/pcd16.180641

[67] Røe Y, Torbjørnsen A, Stanghelle B, Helseth S, Riiser K. Health literacy in higher education: A systematic scoping review of educational approaches. Pedagogy in Health Promotion. 2023;**11**(1):20-29. DOI: 10.1177/23733799231191107

[68] Ubbes VA, Black JM, Ausherman JA. Teaching for understanding in health education: The role of critical and creative thinking skills within constructivism theory. American Journal of Health Education. 1999;**30**(2):67

[69] Ubbes VA, Ausherman JA. Oral-language development in university classrooms: Building health communication through a constructivist theoretical framework. The International Journal of Interdisciplinary Educational Studies. 2022;**17**(2):1. DOI: 10.18848/2327-011X/CGP

[70] Jonassen DH, Campbell JP, Davidson ME. Learning with media: Restructuring the debate. Educational Technology Research and Development. 1994;**42**:31-39. DOI: 10.1007/BF02299089

[71] Efthymiou A, Kalaitzaki A, Kondilis B, Rovithis M. Health literacy continuing education courses and tools for healthcare professionals: A scoping review. Gerontology & Geriatrics Education. 2024;**45**(2):212-247. DOI: 10.1080/02701960.2022.2156865

[72] Champlin S, Hoover DS, Mackert M. Health literacy in adult education centers: Exploring educator and staff needs. Health Promotion Practice. 2020;**21**(2):198-208. DOI: 10.1177/1524839918789690

[73] Barari N, RezaeiZadeh M, Khorasani A, Alami F. Designing and validating educational standards for E-teaching in virtual learning environments (VLEs), based on revised Bloom's taxonomy. Interactive Learning Environments. 2022;**30**(9):1640-1652. DOI: 10.1080/10494820.2020.1739078

[74] Baxter Magolda MB. Self-authorship: The foundation for twenty-first-century education. New Directions for Teaching & Learning. 2007;**2007**(109):69-83. Available from: https://search-ebscohost-com.proxy.lib.miamioh.edu/login.aspx?direct=true&db=aph&AN=24746901&site=ehost-live&scope=site

[75] Hacker DJ, Keener MC, Kircher JC. 9 writing is applied metacognition. In: Handbook of Metacognition in Education. Milton Park, Oxfordshire, UK: Routledge; 2009. pp. 154-172

Chapter 8

Embracing Social Media Trends: Use of Short-Form Videos in Medical Education

Kevlian Andrew, Mary C. Maj and Sharmila Upadhya

Abstract

The aim of the chapter is to highlight the current trends of short-form videos on different social media platforms and how this presents an opportunity for use in medical education. Students are regularly assigned faculty-created videos and readings as part of their directed learning curriculum. These can range from 5 minutes to an hour and are not often well received. Short-form videos are generally 1-2 minutes long and used by many industries to market products or spread information. The younger generations are becoming increasingly familiar with this type of media and can spend hours a day scrolling through these videos on various social media platforms. This chapter will describe a proposal for using short-form videos as a method of content delivery that could potentially have better student reception and perhaps knowledge retention. Despite commercially available videos, faculty development in creating videos can allow for learner-specific customization of content.

Keywords: short-form videos, medical education, knowledge retention, content delivery, learner-specific customization

1. Introduction

From preschool educators to medical school professors, faculty frequently engage in discussions on students' struggles with what would feel like simple concepts from their perspective. Considerations of whether students in professional programs, such as medical school, carefully read the PowerPoint slide packets, looked at the posted video(s), or were attentive during lectures, often arising in attempts to understand the disconnect. Phrases like "all they need to know is..." or "once they understand this..." best summarize the sentiments of faculty's desire for students to know the basic concepts that underpin more complex ideas. However, the newer generations are being introduced to mobile devices and digital tools at increasingly younger ages. As such, they are much more tech-savvy seekers of instant gratification who do not have the natural inclination toward textbook reading assignments or sitting through boring lectures [1–3]. This is a departure from the preferences of educators who prefer textbooks and lecture notes over the Internet for their own learning [4].

Using the generally accepted birth year definitions of generations, Generation Z (1995–2010) is characterized as being the first to have access to digital tools at a very young age. They are considered to be socially liberal, tolerant, innovative, goal-oriented, and technologically inclined. In 2025, the age range of this generation is 15–30 years. Generation Alpha (2010–2025) was born into technology like iPhones and artificial intelligence and has mastered the skill of navigating different apps. They are characterized by their tech-savvy, digital literacy, as well as their optimism, curiosity, self-determination, impatience, and technological dependence [1, 5, 6]. In 2025, their age range is 15 years and under.

Over the past 5 years, the average age of medical students has been 23 years, with most students falling first into the 23–25-year age group, and second, into the 20- to 22-year age bracket [7]. The current and future medical school populations therefore consist of Generation Z (Gen Z), with Generation Alpha (Gen Alpha) set to make their appearance at medical school in 2030. If the present statistics hold true, the medical student population in the 2030s will be comprised of the younger portion of Generation Z (2005–2010) and the older cohort of Generation Alpha (2010–2020).

Considering the familiarity of these two generations with technology, social media, and the boost in technology use following the COVID-19 pandemic [1, 6], attempts to incorporate aspects of their generational norm into medical education may be more achievable than efforts in "forcing" them to conform to traditional educational methods. This chapter briefly discusses the current trends of social media usage of the present and upcoming generations of medical students and explores the possibility of embracing their current habits by leveraging social media tools to promote student engagement in medical education.

2. Methods

The underlying premise of this perspective chapter is the steady increase in the use of social media, especially by the younger generations due to their affinity to technology. As such, a cursory search of the literature on Google Scholar was conducted using the following key phrases: |"educational" AND "needs" AND "generation alpha" AND "generation Z" –"early education" –"gamification" –"childhood education"|, |"social media" AND ("different generations" OR "generation alpha") |and |"short-form videos" AND "impact" AND "attention" AND "generation"|. Time limits were set for literature published from 2016 to 2025. The default setting to 'sort by relevance" was used, and results beyond page 10 were automatically excluded. Articles were excluded if they were topic-specific (e.g., referencing physics/math) or outside the focus of the study (e.g., social media and tourism). Only papers with a focus on Generation Alpha and Generation Z and their educational needs, as well as their social media use and impacts of short-form videos, were further reviewed for more information. Additional key phrase searches were briefly reviewed for the "next generation of medical students" and to gain insight into the historical context of social media ("history of social media platforms"). A regular Google search was used to find simple, "how-to" steps for creating short-form videos ("how to make short-form videos"), as this information was not readily found on Google Scholar.

DOI: http://dx.doi.org/10.5772/intechopen.1010322

3. Background

3.1 Educational needs of generation Z and alpha

Studies show that Generation Z expects an educational format as digitally enhanced as their daily environments. Given their familiarity with readily accessing information *via* technology, and their ability to learn almost anything without conventional instruction, their engagement is maintained by teaching in accordance with their preference of learning through real-life scenarios. As such, adapting lecture content to mirror life cases, along with opportunities for personalized access to online course material (based on convenience, pace, and need for revision), and guidance in navigating digital resources, is recommended. Didactic lectures and textbook readings are therefore considered long and boring in comparison with the already accessible informal resources. These highly visual learners, by virtue of their time spent viewing and interacting with videos and pictures on their devices, require learning resources that more closely align with their way of communication—graphics, animations, videos, and lighthearted humor. The charisma of teachers is reportedly more relevant now than in the past. Leveraging this in flipped classroom settings where students do independent e-learning (prior to class) and then actively engage with content under faculty supervision (in class) has shown to be effective with this generation. Because of their decreasing and distributed attention span over numerous simultaneous tasks, smaller, more meaningful, bite-sized chunks of interactive learning are preferred [3, 8].

Similarly, given their birth into a world of rapidly advancing technology, technology means the world to Generation Alpha [5]. Unlike prior generations that view technology as a tool, digital devices are perceived as a necessity for Generation Alpha. Parents of this generation have reported upwards of 7 hours of daily screen time on mobile devices [4]. Like Gen Z, Gen Alpha requires innovative teaching methods due to their quick access to vast information. A shift toward knowledge development and interpretation, as opposed to information access and delivery, would be crucial. Experiential learning through investigation, experimentation, problem-solving, and creativity capitalizes on their childhood experiences with navigating gadgets, apps, and gaming. They will likely benefit from visual, aural, and kinesthetic digital teaching methods that engage their curiosity and creativity while still developing necessary skills (e.g., reading and critical thinking) [9]. As such, strategically incorporating short-form videos (discussed later), a medium well known to these two generations, may see an increase in student willingness to, and satisfaction with, interacting with learning material.

The ability to meet these technological needs will be hinged on the technological expertise of faculty. Not only have educators struggled to keep abreast of technology, but their perception of the important role played by technology, and the impact of social media on the lives of the younger generations, is also crucial. Faculty who viewed social media as an innovative tool, important to the lives and future happiness of their students, were more likely to integrate this tool into their teaching activities. Conversely, faculty who were older and held the belief that social media is irrelevant to their teaching were less likely to integrate it into their learning materials, even after training on how to do so [4]. Integrating technology would therefore require at least some measure of open-mindedness and flexibility on the part of faculty.

3.2 Social media and current trends

3.2.1 Social media

As the name suggests, social media refers to Internet-based applications that facilitate content creation and sharing and social interactions among its users. The existence of this social software dates to around the 2000s [10, 11]. While older social media platforms such as Friendster and MySpace emerged in 2003, later platforms like Facebook (2004), YouTube (2005), Twitter (2006), and LinkedIn (2009) came about later and are still well known today. The more recent and frequently used additions include Pinterest, Instagram, and WhatsApp which launched in 2010, and Snapchat and WeChat in 2011. These later platforms have capitalized on the use of mobile Internet for the sharing of images and short-form videos. A more recent social media platform, TikTok [12], debuted first in 2016 as Douyin in China and then internationally as TikTok a year later. The different platforms contain a variety of modes for individuals to engage with content and each other including text-only content like chats [13], photos, and videos [12, 13]. It should be noted that in addition to connecting users, social platforms and the entities that use them as a marketplace profit off of user engagement as they work toward user growth and retention [12]. As such, their ability to gain and keep the attention of [12] users by evoking emotional responses is crucial.

3.2.2 Current social media trends

With the most frequently used digital communication tools being mobile devices and apps, the trend of media consumption has been growing for Generation Z and Alpha [1]. The Common Sense Census of 2021 showed an increase in the time spent on social media between 2015 and 2021, with a larger increase seen in the 2 years following the pandemic than observed in the 4 years prior. Using the ages as a proxy for generations, the media usage for members of Generation Z (teens: 13 to 18 years old) increased from 6.67 hours a day in 2015 to 7.37 hours a day in 2019 and 8.65 in 2021. Media time per day for Generation Alpha (tweens: 8 to 12 years old) increased from 4.6 hours in 2015 to 4.73 hours per day in 2019 and 5.55 in 2021. The top 4 most used platforms for watching online videos were YouTube (24%), TikTok (22%), Snapchat (21%), and Instagram (15%).

The increases in time were attributed to time spent watching online videos and using social media platforms. There was a 5% decrease in reading for enjoyment among tweens, but no notable difference in teen reading habits, between 2019 and 2021. Nonetheless, the average reading time per day was 29 to 30 minutes [2]. Even more interesting, the 2020 Common Sense Census on media use by children eight and under showed an average of 2.4 hours of screen media per day [14]. This group of Generation Alpha will begin entering the medical student population in the 2030s.

One TikTok-specific study showed that young people between the ages of 11 and 30 years use the app daily. Most (67.92%) responses came from Generation Z (age 19 to 24 years) working students, 40.57% of whom prefer using the app mostly in the evening and 17.92% mostly at night. It was largely used for entertainment purposes. Most preferred short videos were 1 minute (59.43%) or 15 seconds (30.19%) long. Accordingly, the impatience and desire for concise content were also evident. There was a 74.53% preference for videos with post-production editing that eliminated hesitations and pauses, and a 76.42% preference for videos where there is only the creator speaking directly to the point. After comedic content, educational content was most preferred [15].

3.3 Short-form videos and platforms

Short-form videos are usually brief videos that range from 15 seconds to up to a few minutes long, hence the name [16, 17]. They are typically concise, engaging, and used for the bite-sized delivery of content [17]. As no universal standard for the length exists, these can usually go up to 3 minutes but are generally shorter than 10 minutes. Most platforms have micro videos, which are short videos that run for a few seconds up to a minute [18, 19]. They are typically vertical with a 9:16 aspect ratio, ideal for viewing on mobile devices [20], in contrast to the 16:9 aspect ratio typical of long-form videos. Long-form videos, like those seen on YouTube or the videos commonly seen on learning platforms, last 10 or more minutes. These are best suited for in-depth explanations of topics [17, 18].

Short-form videos are currently found on almost all social media platforms. They were introduced in 2020 on platforms like Vines and Muscical.ly, the former which went away and the latter which was bought and relaunched into the notorious original short-form app, TikTok [21]. Short-form videos later became incorporated into other platforms: Instagram (reels – 2019, stories and posts), YouTube (shorts), Facebook (reels, stories and posts), and WhatsApp (statuses) [11, 13, 18, 21]. TikTok, specifically, is a short-form video app, with 15-second video allowances for common users and 60-second video allowances for viewers with larger followings [13]. Instagram reels range from 15 to 90 seconds, and YouTube and Snapchat videos go up to 60 seconds [17]. The popularity of this type of media is partially due to their ability to cater to the decreasing attention span of humans [17, 19].

3.4 Impact of short-form videos

Previous studies have shown that exposure to the increasing number of stimuli through online content decreases one's ability to pay attention. This is attributed to the shared volume of content that the mind is exposed to and must therefore process. The human attention span has been shown to decline from 12 seconds to 8 seconds, 1 second less endurance than that of a goldfish [15].

As a result of the increased engagement in social media, not only has concentration and attention been impaired, but also social media addiction has emerged. This has been described as the inability to go without opening the application, even for a brief second [15]. Binge-scrolling of short-form videos, a behavior that emerged during the COVID-19 pandemic, has also become a concern. One study showed that participants spent a daily average of 2.26 hours scrolling through short-form videos, most commonly in the evening or later at night. The motivating factors included entertainment, escapism, and coping with stress. Despite the negative outcomes of procrastination, negative emotions, and decreased sleep, some neutral outcomes of scrolling included learning new information and online socialization [16].

Social network systems can motivate users' behaviors through their ability to satisfy different user needs and thus provide gratification. Motivating factors with the strongest correlation to watching TikTok videos included seeking novelty (learning new things) and because of habit. However, both the proportion of positive feedback users received and the degree of loneliness they felt positively correlated with the length of time they spent on the app. Passive use of the app (i.e., consuming content without creating and uploading) has also been shown to both negatively and positively correlate with user well-being. This was dependent on the user's motivation for watching the short-from videos, that is, positive motivations correlated with positive outcomes [13].

It should also be noted that Generation Alpha's early introduction to social media has raised some questions about its impact on their social-emotional development [4]. With their social interaction being driven by their consumption of digital media, concerns over the loss of skills like oral communication (due to constant texting) and critical thinking (due to reliance on social media for learning) have surfaced. Some have also found decreased self-esteem and higher levels of anxiety in young children with extended exposure to "virtual leisure" and limited social interactions with people. However, it is believed that these effects can be mitigated through engagement with adults. This includes parents who are involved in their children's lives, and trained teachers who are knowledgeable about technology and can guide this generation in effectively engaging with it through their teaching [4].

4. Short-form video use in medical education

4.1 Creating short-from videos: Content

Considering the digital nature of Generation Z and Alpha and their consumption of short-form videos, coupled with the declining attention spans [15], an opportunity to incorporate this natural, and increasingly pervasive, behavior presents itself for medical educators. Users have been shown to stick around for 70% of videos under 2 minutes, with engagement decreasing as video length increased to 3 to 5 minutes [22]. Presenting the same material in a more concise and interesting format could improve the chances that students would remain engaged for a larger proportion of a 2- to 3-minute video compared to engagement for a 50-minute lecture [19]. Short-form videos check the boxes of providing digital content that can be conveniently accessed, providing bite-sized information that can be progressively built upon over time, representing real-life scenarios, and promoting engagement [3, 8].

4.1.1 Topic selection

User-preferred content ideas that best fit the educational format include quick tips, tutorials, how-to's, and animated explainers. These are meant to educate the audience, teach useful skills and tasks, and simplify complex topics [17, 18]. As these videos are "short," care and attention must be paid to selecting the topic. As they cannot be too broad, for example, "Anatomy of the Upper Limb," "Lipoproteins" or "Central Dogma of Molecular Biology," narrower subtopics should be selected to fit within the time frame. More suitable examples of topics that address the anatomy of the upper limb include "Muscles of the Arm," "Muscles of the Anterior Forearm," and "Muscles of the Hand." Likewise, the broad topic of "Lipoproteins" can be divided into key elements such as "Chylomicron Metabolism" and "VLDL and LDL metabolism." Similarly, the broad topic of "Central dogma of molecular biology" can be divided into key components such as "Origin of DNA Replication" and "Transcription of protein-coding genes." Consideration should also be given to the target student group and their prior knowledge level. A short-form video that may be appropriate for second-year medical students who have already covered the basics of the body systems may not work for first-year students who would not have yet received the introductory/foundational information. Similarly, a video to be viewed before starting a new topic would likely cover basic concepts versus one placed after covering that topic, which could now be more intricate. As such, the placement of the video within the curriculum should also be carefully considered [8].

4.1.2 Objectives

The objectives to be covered in the video would again be dictated by the length of the video. One video can potentially cover one complex or higher-order objective, or a few simpler, lower-order objectives. For example, a short-form video on the "Muscles of the Arm" can (1) Describe the compartments of the arm, (2) Describe the general action, and innervation of the muscles of the compartments of the arm, and (3) Identify the muscles of the arm—three lower-order objectives. This would also be a good example of a video found toward the start of a series of lectures on the muscles of the upper limb. Conversely, if the same topic were covered toward the end of the upper limb anatomy series, a video of the same length could cover a more complex objective like a real-life case involving trauma to the arm and analysis of the resulting deficits [3, 8].

4.1.3 Script and content

The topic and associated objectives would inform the outline or script that would be required for the video. An attention grabber should be placed within the first 3 seconds of the video [20]. This can be done using catchy visuals, compelling statements, or intriguing questions. For the rest of the video, storytelling is shown to be a good way to create engaging videos [17, 19]. The biggest challenge would be condensing explanations of the objectives (or "stories") down to a few sentences that would fit the time limit. A helpful way to go about creating a script would be to ask, "What *must* the student walk away from this video knowing or understanding?" Anything that is not an absolute necessity based on the answer to this question can be communicated to the students in some other way. Cramming too much into a video or going too fast can become overwhelming [8, 19] and should therefore be avoided. A word-for-word script may not be necessary if an outline is sufficient to complete the task [22].

The hook sandwich theory (using a hook, delivering content, and using a hook again) [19] can be considered for the videos tending toward the lengthier side of the short-form video spectrum. If necessary, a series of videos can be created to deliver the story in parts [17]. This can accommodate shortened attention spans [15] while facilitating the breakdown of larger concepts into their basic parts. It also affords the opportunity for creating content that progressively builds upon itself, video by video [8]. For example, one short-form video about the "Muscles of the Arm" could be further split into smaller videos addressing each arm compartment individually or begin with the bones and subsequently layer in the arteries, nerves, and then muscles of the different compartments as the series progresses. Moving through this series can be likened to scrolling through different videos on social media. A call to action in the context of social media encourages engagement with the content by asking users to comment, like, or share a video. In the education context, a call to action toward an associated activity (e.g., quiz or case questions, activity sheet, or some other learning activity) could also encourage engagement [18].

Further information can also be provided as a brief description associated with the video, a text box comment on the video, or as part of an activity associated with the video. This leads to the importance of considerations about the format and type of visuals to be used in the video [22]. Some short-form videos simply contain a video of the speaker talking through the narrative, similar to a video recording of a lecture. This is a good start, as user preference has been shown for such videos where the creator speaks directly to the consumer and gets straight to the point [15]. Subtitles improve accessibility by allowing the viewing of content without sound (e.g., for those with hearing impairment or those who prefer soundless viewing) [17, 19].

Narrative videos can be complemented by background still image(s) or video(s) that visually depict what is being described or explained. These can remain the same throughout the entirety of the video or they can be changed based on what is being said. The background visuals can be directly referenced by the speaker at strategic places while they narrate the video. These should be simple and clear and facilitate understanding of the narrative. Alternatively, the video of the presenter can be omitted, leaving only the visuals and the accompanying audio. An alternative is to record a voiceover to go along with b-roll, for example., a recording of someone performing the range of motion on a joint could be accompanied by a voiceover explaining the movements and the muscles that are acting on the joint to produce them [22].

As the attraction of short videos, despite the decreasing attention span, is due to the structure and editing of the videos [15], the additional feature of text box write-ups can be leveraged in different ways. These can promote engagement as the audience reads along as the video plays. They can remain visible for as long as they are set to display. Outside of being used in conjunction with narrative videos, it is also common to see some short-form videos with text boxes overlaying visuals and background music without any narrative audio. This can potentially translate well into the educational context when considering videos like animations about the process of DNA replication or coagulation cascade.

4.2 Creating short-form videos: Production

On the most basic level, all that is necessary for the creation of a short-form video is a device with video recording capabilities, that is, a device with a camera, a microphone, and a speaker (like a phone). Resultantly, most of the content that is produced and uploaded to social media is filmed and edited on a mobile device, a common commodity [22]. As such, the initial cost for anyone desiring to make short-form videos would most likely surround the purchase of software to access more advanced editing features. It should be noted, however, that the type and features of the phone would dictate the quality of the video that can be produced.

Before filming, ensure that all necessary equipment, props, and visual aids (e.g., tools like whiteboard and markers) [20] are present by reviewing the objectives and script and creating a list of all that would be necessary to tell the desired story. Considerations of recording location should include a quiet space with good lighting and little to no echo or background noises, or potential for disruption. Positioning of subjects would depend on the audiovisual devices being used and the setup (e.g., filming from a phone on a tripod vs. filming at a desktop). Regardless, testing the setup to ensure good audio and visuals should be done before beginning the recording process [22]. Although short-form videos are typically filmed vertically (9:16 aspect ratio), this is not necessarily a requirement. However, this is one of the optimizations for mobile viewing and should be given serious consideration since mobiles are the most frequently used device for viewing online content [17, 19].

Faculty need not start from scratch as there is also the option of repurposing long-form content such as previous lectures or other video recordings. Snippets from these can be taken and enhanced with editing for conversion into short-form videos [19, 21]. Once the topic(s) has been selected, the objectives are chosen, and the desired content (e.g., visuals and/or audio) is identified, the creation process can begin. Whether recording new content or repurposing old ones, it would be helpful to schedule in time to accomplish these tasks. After the first couple of attempts, faculty will learn how to budget their time to produce these videos. Having a good idea of where in the lesson plan these videos would be placed, similar to a social media posting schedule, will also assist with the scheduling process for production planning.

The most important task would be the editing of the video [18], which allows for the removal of excess footage and the addition of the features that users find engaging, that is, combinations of sounds, text, images, and post-production enhancements [15, 22]. Some social media platforms and other software have simple tools that can assist with the editing process. Recommendations for beginners include using the original sound, adding sound effects or music, and adding text overlays that can be used to highlight key points [18, 20, 22]. Commonly used, simple editing tools include Canva, CapCut, Kapwing, InShot, iMove, Quik by GoPro, Magisto, and Clipomatic. Examples of more advanced software include Kinemaster and Adobe Premiere Rush [18, 22]. As the editing features would be unique to the recording and/or editing software, it would be important for faculty to become familiarized with the specific tools available to them.

4.3 Faculty training and resources

Faculty training would be a requirement to successfully create and deliver content using short-form videos. It is known that as members of prior, less digital generations, faculty may not be as technologically adept as the Gen Z and Gen Alpha digital natives [9]. Without such training, educators are unable to be responsive to the digital inclinations of the younger generations. Providing faculty with the necessary support, time, and resources, including personalized training that would address the specific characteristics and needs of the educator, would be an important consideration. However, a key component in successfully implementing such a change would be gauging the current perception of faculty regarding the use of short-form videos. Faculty resistance to integrating this tool, regardless of training, is unlikely to yield results [4].

Since the COVID-19 pandemic forced the world into distance learning [9], most institutions likely use faculty-created videos in their curriculum. As such, the basic materials for creating videos may already be in place: devices with cameras, and programs for recording and editing videos. If making a new recording, the simplest way to start the transition toward using short-form videos would be for faculty to create videos in the same way they normally would, using the resources they are familiar with but limiting the time to a few minutes. The required resources would therefore be whatever the institution already uses, which would also make for easier integration of videos into the existing learning management systems. Alternatively, repurposing already existing long-form videos would likely be the quickest method of producing short-form videos without the effort of creating from scratch [19].

Drawing on prior experience with recording and performing basic editing of online videos, the training could potentially be centered around the editing functions specific to short-form videos—the addition of text boxes, background images, or videos and adjusting the audio overlay, if used [18, 19]. Training in how to use editing features would need to be specific to the software made available by the institution for faculty use. Alternatively, other existing programs that have been designed specifically for creating social media content, with free and paid versions, can be used to assist with the creation of these videos [18, 22]. Learning how to use the different software would likely require additional training for most faculty who may not be familiar with these tools. When using such tools, as they are designed specifically for social media, consideration needs to be given to the compatibility of the institution's video delivery platform (learning management system) with the created 9:16 short-form video and the video uploading process.

It should be mentioned that the capacity of artificial intelligence tools to generate scripts and images holds considerable promise in generating the content for short-form video creation a little less daunting. Institutions also have the option to outsource short-form video editing and or creation. Given the dominance of social media marketing, companies have emerged that capitalize on providing such services [17, 19]. If possible, institutions could also look into diversifying their employee roster to include personnel with the technical know-how for creating and editing short-form videos for in-house production and customization [9]. Medical illustrators would be an example of such personnel.

Implementation of all the above would undoubtedly require time to not only procure resources and offer faculty training but also gain their buy-in for any efforts to yield results. While Generation Z currently forms a portion of the medical student population and may benefit from this initiative, medical educators still have just about 5 years before the more digitally native Generation Alpha matriculate into medical schools. This provides some time for institutions, and their faculty, to weigh their options and potentially start reviewing current curricula and resources for ideas [18] on creating short-form videos.

4.4 Suggested uses

The use of short-form videos is not meant to replace lectures or reading assignments but can be used to augment these teaching activities. Converting one 20-minute lecture into the short-form video format would probably require at least six videos, depending on the length and editing of the short-form video [18]. While this may naturally improve the engagement of younger generations, given their shorter attention spans, the intention should be to design content that prioritizes both engagement and interaction of all learners over information delivery. As an example, a lecture can be converted to a flipped classroom where pre-assignments include short-form videos along with questions/activity worksheets that can be expanded upon during the lecture. Repurposing a lecture to create short-form videos could therefore serve as an opportunity to capitalize on this focus as opposed to simply delivering the same information in shorter videos.

Short-form videos can also be associated with a block of practice questions to highlight the common key concept being tested in the series of questions. While leveraging the direct, to-the-point narrative aspect of short-form videos, these can also assist faculty with providing rationales for a group of questions as opposed to generating individual question rationales. They also allow faculty to provide interactive ("face-to-face"), guided summaries of applied concepts that students can access on their own. The use of mini-case short-form videos can also facilitate the provision of real-life scenarios that the younger generations need to appreciate the relevance of what they are learning. A case can unfold in phases throughout a series of videos, with the time in between used for students to reflect on and apply concepts before moving forward. Faculty must embrace the notion that technology is not just a tool but a lived experience for the younger generations. This should thus be leveraged in providing the experiential learning to which they have grown accustomed.

4.5 Mitigating negative effects

While the motivations for watching short-from videos are linked to the outcomes (i.e., a positive correlation between positive motivations and positive outcomes) [13], the correlation between screen time and negative outcomes cannot be ignored [15]. Excessive consumption of short-form videos has been linked to behavioral and psychological issues, like emotional dysregulation, poor sleep, poor concentration and attention, and decreased time management [16]. Although the suggestion is to leverage a tool that the younger generations are already familiar with, the conscientious use of short-form videos to avoid encouraging addictive behaviors is key. Limiting the amount of screen time would therefore need to be a consideration when creating and integrating short-form videos into the curriculum. However, further research is needed to assess the impact of educational/curricular-based short-form videos on addictive tendencies to gain better insight into quantifying the ideal time limit.

Additionally, it is important to highlight that despite the ability of social media and short-form videos to engage the younger generations, there is no substitute for the skills learned through in-person interactions [4]. As such, short-form video usage should not be used to replace lectures or in person teaching, but as a tool to augment these interactive sessions. Maintaining this perspective can reduce the risk of creating excessive amounts of short-form videos. It also ensures that the videos are not provided as independent resources but as supplemental tools associated with live, interactive sessions. Prioritizing use of these tools to design team-based and problem-based session sessions could also help faulty to guide Generation Alpha in developing skills like critical thinking, collaboration, and communication [6].

5. Limitations and considerations

Due to time constraints, short-form videos limit how much information can be conveyed in one video. Based on their placement in the curriculum, they can be used for sharing basic, foundational concepts before starting more complex topics, or they can be used after a topic has been covered to review salient points or encourage the application of knowledge. As with most things, not all individuals in the medical student population may gravitate toward this tool. According to the AAMC data, if the proportions do not change significantly, it can be expected that around 25% of the class in the 2030s will come from Generation Alpha (those born in 2010) [1, 7]. This leaves the remaining portion coming from Generation Z, who will likely still appreciate this approach, and non-traditional students from prior generations.

Technology and trends consistently change and the social media platforms in existence today may evolve or may not be as commonly used by 2030. As such, exposure and training in the use of short-form videos should therefore be focused on the features that have been shown to improve engagement with Gen Z and Gen Alpha, as opposed to the specific features of the different platforms.

6. Conclusion

During the 2030s, the population of medical students will comprise the latter groups of Generation Z and the earlier portion of Generation Alpha. Current data shows that these generations have an affinity for the technology that shaped their upbringing and can spend hours a day scrolling through social media. While this has been shown to have negative impacts on attention span and emotions, interacting with the world through technology is a way of normal existence for the younger generations. This presents an opportunity for faculty to use the same technology to meet students where they are in their lived, digital context. Short-form videos can accommodate the decreasing attention spans of the younger generations while still achieving the purpose of learning through experience and engagement. This would require faculty to shift their focus from information delivery to promoting active engagement and real-life learning through leveraging technology to achieve these goals. The changing needs of the students, regardless of improvements in technology or influence by social media and/or trends, will continue to inspire educators to seek new and improved ways to teach students in all levels of education.

Conflict of interest

The authors declare no conflict of interest.

Author details

Kevlian Andrew[1], Mary C. Maj[2] and Sharmila Upadhya[2*]

1 School of Medicine, Anatomical Sciences, St. George's University, True Blue, St. George, Grenada

2 Department of Biochemistry, St. George's University, School of Medicine, True Blue, St. George, Grenada

*Address all correspondence to: shupadhya@sgu.edu

References

[1] Šramova B, Pavelka J. Transgenerational Approach Focused on Generation Z and Generation Alpha to Current Consumption of Mobile Applications [Internet]. Dykinson: Torrossa; 2023. Available from: https://www.torrossa.com/en/resources/an/5577486 [Accessed: January 18, 2025]

[2] Rideout V, Robb MB, Mann S, Peebles A. The Common Sense Census: Media Use by Tweens and Teens, 2021 [Internet]. Common Sense Media. Common Sense; 2022 [cited 2025 Jan 19]. Available from: https://www.commonsensemedia.org/research/the-common-sense-census-media-use-by-tweens-and-teens-2021

[3] Cretu I, Grigore M, Scripcariu I-S. Get ready for gen Z, our next generation of medical students. Revista de Cercetare si Interventie Sociala. 2020;**69**:283-292

[4] Höfrová A, Balidemaj V, Small MA. A systematic literature review of education for generation alpha. Discover Education. [Internet]. 15 Aug 2024;**3**(125) [cited 2025 Jan 12]. Available from: https://link.springer.com/article/10.1007/s44217-024-00218-3

[5] Jha AK. Understanding generation alpha [Internet]. 20 Jun 2020 [cited 2025 Jan 12]. Available from: https://osf.io/preprints/osf/d2e8g_v1

[6] Drugas M. Screenagers or "Screamagers"? Current perspectives on generation alpha. Psychological Thought. 2022;**15**(1):1-11

[7] Matriculating Student Questionnaire (MSQ) [Internet]. AAMC; 2024 [cited 2025 Jan 12]. Available from: https://www.aamc.org/data-reports/students-residents/report/matriculating-student-questionnaire-msq

[8] Lerchenfeldt S, Attardi SM, Pratt RL, Sawarynski KE, Taylor TA. Twelve tips for interfacing with the new generation of medical students: Igen. Medical Teacher. 2020;**43**(11):1249-1254

[9] Ziatdinov R, Cilliers J. Generation alpha: Understanding the next cohort of university students. European Journal of Contemporary Education. 18 Sep 2021;**10**(3):783-789

[10] Fietkiewicz KJ, Stock WG, Lins E, Baran KS. Other times, other manners: How do different generations use social media? [Internet]. In: 2016 Hawaii University International Conferences. Arts, Humanities, Social Sciences & Education; 2016. Available from: https://www.academia.edu/39517171/Other_times_other_manners_How_do_different_generations_use_social_media [Accessed: January 18, 2025]

[11] Helmond A, Van der Vlist FN. Social media and platform historiography: Challenges and opportunities. TMG Journal for Media History. 2019;**22**(1):6

[12] Carrigan M, Fatsis L. 2. The history of platforms. In: The Public and their Platforms [Internet]. Bristol, UK: Bristol University Press; 2021. pp. 31-54. [cited 2025 Jan 12]. Available from: https://bristoluniversitypressdigital.com/display/book/9781529201062/ch002.xml

[13] Dong Z, Xie T. Why do people love short-form videos? the motivations for using Chinese tiktok (Douyin) and implications for well-being. Current Psychology [Internet]. 26 Apr 2024;**43**(26):22283-22296. [cited 2025 Jan 12]. Available from: https://www.researchgate.net/publication/380107656_Why_do_people_love_short-form_videos_The_

motivations_for_using_Chinese_TikTok_Douyin_and_implications_for_well-being

[14] Rideout V, Robb MB. The Common Sense Census: Media Use by Kids Age Zero to Eight, 2020 [Internet]. Common Sense Media. Common Sense; 2020 [cited 2025 Jan 19]. Available from: https://www.commonsensemedia.org/research/the-common-sense-census-media-use-by-kids-age-zero-to-eight-2020

[15] Tirendi D, Gargiulo L. Measuring the impacts of social media on daily life from millennials to generation alpha. International Journal of Research in Humanities and Social Studies. 2024;**11**(3):26-33

[16] Xu S. Exploring short-form videos binge-scrolling behaviors among college students [thesis]. ProQuest Dissertations & Theses; 2024

[17] Hareem. How to Make Short-form Video Content that Stands Out in 2025 [Internet]. ContentStudio; 2024 [cited 2025 Jan 19]. Available from: https://contentstudio.io/blog/how-to-make-short-form-video-content

[18] Frink-DeLary S. A Guide to Creating Short-Form Video Content [Internet]. Real Marketing Solutions; 2024. Available from: https://realmarketingsolutions.net/how-to-create-short-form-video-content/ [Accessed: January 19, 2025]

[19] Shieldsmith J. The Ultimate Guide to Short-Form Video (Trends, Tips, and More!) [Internet]. The Ultimate Guide to Short-form Video (Trends, Tips, and More!). Available from: https://www.veed.io/learn/short-form-video; [Accessed: January 19, 2025]

[20] Meyer TT. 52 Short-Form Video Tips [Internet]. StrongMocha; 2025. Available from: https://strongmocha.com/beginners-guides/52-short-form-video-tips/ [Accessed: January 19, 2025]

[21] West C. The Ultimate Guide to Short-Form Video Content [Internet]. Influencer Marketing Hub; 2024. Available from: https://influencermarketinghub.com/short-form-video-content/ [Accessed: January 19, 2025]

[22] Bonacci J. How to Make a Short Video: Your Comprehensive Guide [Internet]. WebFX; 2023. Available from: https://www.webfx.com/blog/content-marketing/how-to-make-a-short-video/ [Accessed: January 19, 2025]